Balancing Act
The New Medical Ethics of Medicine's New Economics

CLINICAL MEDICAL ETHICS

Editors

Previous Books in the Series

Balancing Act
The New Medical Ethics of Medicine's New Economics

E. Haavi Morreim

GEORGETOWN UNIVERSITY PRESS / WASHINGTON, D.C.

To Florence and Paul,
my mother and father,
with all my love.

Georgetown University Press, Washington, D.C.
© 1995 by Georgetown University Press. All rights reserved.
Printed in the United States of America
10 9 8 7 6 5 4 3 2 1   1995
THIS VOLUME IS PRINTED ON ACID-FREE OFFSET BOOK PAPER

Library of Congress Cataloging-in-Publication Data

Morreim, E. Haavi.
    Balancing act : the new medical ethics of medicine's new economics
/ E. Haavi Morreim.
        p.   cm.
    Includes bibliographical references and index.
    1. Medical care—Cost control—Moral and ethical aspects.
    2. Managed care plans (Medical care)—Moral and ethical aspects.
    3. Health care rationing—Moral and ethical aspects.   4. Physician
and patient.   I. Title.
RA410.5.M667   1995
174'.26—dc20
ISBN 0-87840-584-4   94-37058

Contents

Acknowledgments   vii

Notice   viii

1 Overview   1
NOTES   6

2 A Bit of History   8
SOURCES OF COST ESCALATION   9
EARLY EFFORTS AT COST CONTAINMENT   13
FUTURE ECONOMIC PRESSURES   15
NOTES   17

3 Economic Forces, Clinical Constraints   21
BROAD ECONOMIC FORCES   21
INSTITUTIONAL PAYERS AND PROVIDERS   23
CLINICAL CONSTRAINTS   29
SUMMARY   37
NOTES   38

4 Fiscal Scarcity: Challenging Fidelity   43
TRADITIONAL CONCEPTS OF FIDELITY   43
FISCAL SCARCITY   47
CHALLENGING FIDELITY   51
SUMMARY   63
NOTES   65

5   The Limits and Obligations of
    Fidelity: Resource Use   69
    THE LIMITS OF FIDELITY   69
    THE OBLIGATIONS OF FIDELITY   85
    CONCLUSION   98
    NOTES   99

6   The Obligations and Limits of Fidelity:
    Physicians' Professional Services   103
    THE OBLIGATIONS OF FIDELITY   104
    THE LIMITS OF FIDELITY   123
    NOTES   128

7   The New Medical Ethics of
    Medicine's New Economics   131
    AUTONOMY AS FREEDOM   131
    AUTONOMY AS RESPONSIBILITY   134
    THE NEW MEDICAL ETHICS   138
    CONCLUSION   147
    NOTES   148

    References   155
    BOOKS AND ARTICLES   155
    CASES AND STATUTES   175

    Index   177

Acknowledgments

With deep gratitude I acknowledge the colleague-friends who have read portions of this manuscript and shared their valued reflections. They have helped me enormously. They include: Robert Arnold, M.D.; Howard Brody, M.D., Ph.D.; Charles Dougherty, Ph.D.; Howard Entman, M.D.; Peter Jacobson, J.D.; Erich Loewy, M.D.; Thomas Kennedy, Ph.D.; Laurence McCullough, Ph.D.; Charles Pinches, Ph.D.; Michael Rie, M.D.; Lawrence Schneiderman, M.D.; and Margery Shaw, M.D., J.D.

I would particularly like to thank those who have critically reviewed the manuscript in its entirety: Terrence Ackerman, Ph.D.; H. Tristram Engelhardt, Jr., Ph.D., M.D.; Leonard Fleck, Ph.D.; Paul Menzel, Ph.D.; Robert M. Nelson, M.D.; Stuart Spicker, Ph.D.; Stephen Wear, Ph.D.; and several anonymous reviewers. The time, thought, and help they each so generously gave improved this volume immeasurably. While I therefore owe them great credit for its strengths, the book's flaws remain, of course, my own.

And finally, I offer a special and very personal thanks to Tris Engelhardt. He has supported and encouraged my work since I was a graduate student—before I entered this profession, and long before he proposed (in a pub in Sydney, Australia) that I write this volume. Thank you, Tris.

Notice

Except in the instance of cases that have been reported in the public media or have become public through court hearings, all identifiable information used in case examples has been changed, and the structure of the case examples has been altered, so as not to identify the individuals involved. Instead, case examples have been constructed out of numerous clinical experiences so as to illustrate a general problem in bioethics, health care delivery, or health care policy. Any similarity to actual individuals living or dead is purely coincidental.

Also, though legal cases and principles are examined in this volume, there is no intention to provide legal advice. For legal advice there is no substitute for directly subvening the legal profession.

1

Overview

Medicine's changing economics have fundamentally, permanently altered the relationship between physician and patient. Traditionally, that relationship has been dyadic. Physician and patient, usually consulting only with each other or perhaps with family members, would do whatever they thought best. Until fairly recently, the physician had relatively little to offer the patient other than his[1] own personal knowledge, skill, and effort. And as new technologies emerged, third-party payers covered their costs, enabling the physician to continue to focus almost exclusively on the patient. These payers stood not as participating members of the relationship, but mainly as silent partners to finance and facilitate. Although the physician sometimes faced competing obligations, as for instance to other patients or to the patient's family, his professional obligation was overwhelmingly centered on each patient.

For a wide variety of reasons this situation has changed profoundly, as the physician's obligations to each patient are now embedded in a network of competing obligations and conflicting interests. Physicians can no longer deliver adequate care by using only their own knowledge and skill. They commonly must use costly technologies—an array of medical and monetary resources—that usually are owned by other people. These others, having watched their expenditures rise exponentially over the past three decades, are no longer willing to remain silent partners. Those who directly pay for health care, including government, businesses, and insurers, are instituting a broad variety of controls and incentives to ensure that physicians and patients consider the economic as well as the medical wisdom of their plans. In like manner hospitals, clinics, and other institutions that provide technologies and ancillary services are circumscribing more carefully just what facilities they will offer, to whom, under what conditions.

What I will state now, and substantiate later, is that these economic agents who provide and now more closely manage the physical and fiscal resources of care are not intruders[2] into the health care relationship. They are intimately a part of it. If the physician–patient relationship was once a simple dyad, this was only because the times, and medicine itself, were simpler. In the vastly more complex present and future, the physician's obligations to the patient can no longer be a single-minded, unequivocal commitment, but rather must reflect a balancing. Patients' interests must be weighed against the legitimate competing claims of other patients, of payers, of society as a whole, and sometimes even of the physician himself. Although there still is a physician–patient relationship, it is now set within a broader health care nexus. In this latter context, the rights and interests of economic agents, society, and other parties are both routine and proper, not exceptional or per se morally distasteful.

Against this changed setting, we must consider anew just what moral and professional commitment the physician owes, and does not owe, the patient. Equally important, we must also inquire what obligations patients have. I will argue that the physician is not obligated to bypass legitimate contracts or program limits, to ignore other patients' competing interests, or even to efface totally his own interests. Rather, the physician owes his patient what is his to give. He owes some very traditional duties, such as professional competence, compassion, and honesty. And he has some rather new duties, including economic advocacy, economic disclosure, and a close scrutiny of the economic structures and institutions with which he affiliates.

Conversely, I will also argue that patients must assume a new role. Whereas we may be accustomed to thinking only about protecting the patient's freedom to choose as he wishes and act as he pleases, it is now time to expect the patient to exercise responsibility for his own choices not only over individual medical decisions, but also over other matters, such as lifestyle choices and selection of his health care coverage. The patient's active participation in shaping the new economics of health care is not merely to be permitted; it is to be expected.

Throughout this volume I will focus on the clinical setting—on the ethical issues that the new economics of health care poses for physicians in the office, at the bedside, and even on the telephone. I will not attempt to answer broader social questions that, although important, are vigorously debated elsewhere. Thus, I will not inquire whether government ought to fund universal health insurance, or whether health care should be considered a right, or whether all citizens should have equal access to the same quality of care. Rather, I intend to discuss the health care system, not in terms of what it ought one day to be, but in terms of what it is today and in the foreseeable future, and what moral problems our current reality poses for the practicing physician.

Although we[3] will focus on health care in the United States, we can safely say that physicians everywhere are likely to face many of the same basic issues of clinical ethics, quite regardless of the particular system of health care financing and distribution under which they practice. Whether health care is financed by the market or the government, whether providers are public employees or private entrepreneurs, no health care system has enough resources to meet literally every need of every citizen. So long as the physician has the clinical authority to decide what resources to offer which patients, he will inevitably face questions about when to offer "everything" to his own patients and when to accede, and how far, to others' competing claims. And where health resource policies seem unfair or unreasonable, any physician must consider whether to abide by them, or work to change them, or quietly "game the system" to work around them.

Our inquiry will be practical in another way. As the aim of this volume is to address the moral issues that economic changes pose for practicing physicians, I do not intend to engage in metaethical contemplation or even to rely explicitly on theoretical normative reasoning, except where necessary. Rather, the method will be what I call "moral problem-solving." We will focus on the moral problems actually encountered in the clinical practice of medicine, and let these examples frame an analysis that not only affirms and explicates the values we normally bring to our moral dilemmas, but also takes account of the powerful and inevitable complexities and uncertainties that defy any simplistic application of moral principles to real situations. In thus working from 'bottom to top,' the approach will contrast markedly with one particularly popular mode of bioethical reasoning, sometimes known as the 'engineering model' of ethics.[4]

In many textbooks on bioethics it is common to portray a moral issue as a terrible situation in which two or more fundamental moral principles are locked in irreconcilable conflict. The moral agent is then required to find the right normative theory (confirmed as right through a laborious and sophisticated discourse of metaethical reasoning) from which to deduce the morally correct answer to his dilemma. Thus, in a typical hypothetical case, the intensive care unit has only one available bed, while in the emergency room there simultaneously appear four patients needing intensive care: a mother of six, an alcoholic priest, a convicted homicidal rapist, and a brilliant but elderly scientist. The student must decide which one the physician should save, and whom to send back onto the streets to his doom. This philosophical quandary is seen in turn to require one to resort to a broader and more profound metaethical theory, perhaps teleological, deontological, or mixed, from which he can then infer the right resolution.

Interestingly, this approach closely resembles a Newtonian conception of scientific medicine. In this view, medicine is founded on precise and immutable laws of nature that, if we can but discover them fully, will tell us about every part and process of the body. In principle, the physician needs only to apply this general knowledge to the patient's particular situation to deduce the correct diagnosis and therapy. Though he may not always achieve this goal in practice, it is medicine's ideal.[5]

Whether in morals or in medicine, then, it is supposed that at least in principle we can avoid all guesswork, if only we do our homework. In fact, however, this conception does not describe either medicine or morality very well, certainly not in practice and probably not even in principle.[6] Admittedly, the physician can sometimes provide truly Newtonian clinical care. He identifies an infectious organism under the microscope or in a laboratory culture, he understands the natural history of the disease it will cause, and he selects just the right antibiotic to eradicate the organism and cure the disease. Yet much of medicine does not fit this tidy pattern, even in principle. Not all diseases are precisely definable entities with a clearly describable natural history. Patients often do not present as "textbook cases." Their many signs and symptoms may be consistent with a variety of diagnoses, and even after the most thorough workup the physician may be unable to do more than identify the several most likely diagnoses and offer his clinical hunch.[7]

Selecting therapies may be no more precise. Where there are several options, each will have its chances for and against success, and each will have its costs in side effects and inconvenience as well as money. The decision is therefore chosen in light of values, not deduced from certainties.

In sum, medical problem-solving is marked by pervasive uncertainty in which good care results not so much from the physician's technical facility in applying general principles to a particular situation as from his capacity to exercise professional judgment, balancing limited basic principles against practical realities.[8]

Moral problem-solving is remarkably similar. As in medicine, one must first diagnose the problem. And just as medical diagnosis requires information about everything from lab values to the patient's social history, moral diagnostics too can require careful empirical investigation. Issues are not always as they seem. A patient who states that he has religious objections to a particular treatment, for example, might in fact be offering this socially accepted refusal instead of stating his real concern: that he can't afford to pay for the treatment and would be humiliated to accept charity. Until the physician knows what, really, the facts are, he can not determine what, really, is the moral problem—just as in medicine.[9]

And just as in medicine, a fact-careful diagnostic inquiry must be followed by equally practical problem-solving. Our moral lives are comprised, not of terrible hypotheticals from which there is no escape, but of complex situations whose constituent elements are often amenable to considerable alteration. One's moral aim is not ordinarily to undertake a deeply philosophical prioritization of fundamental principles so that he can make dramatic choices that honor one value at a terrible sacrifice of another. Though such sophisticated normative rumination is sometimes required in a truly intractable situation, under ordinary circumstances one's moral aim is rather to forge some resolution that will maximally honor all the important competing values. If the impoverished Jones family vows that they cannot afford to have another child they do not, upon discovering that Mrs. Jones is again pregnant, ask themselves, "Gosh, which of the children shall we throw out onto the streets?" They reconsider the situation and, if they do not consider pregnancy termination to be an option, they decide which things previously regarded as indispensable they will now learn to do without.[10]

As in medicine, uncertainty is often both the driving force and the final remainder. One does not have a dilemma unless there are at least two alternatives, each of which has good reasons on its behalf and serious reasons against it, neither of them clearly preferable to the other. Once again, therefore, a good answer is marked not by some sort of definitive correctness as measured by some clear, precise, objective standard, but rather by the quality of one's reasoning.[11] If one has carefully assembled his facts, conscientiously deliberated about the trade-offs at stake, and creatively forged a resolution that maximally honors the important competing values, we cannot morally ask for better.

This volume will begin with moral diagnostics. Only with a keen factual appreciation of health care's changing economics can we understand the moral conflicts in which physicians find themselves. Those conflicts will emerge as a series of challenges to physicians' traditional fiduciary obligations to hold each patient's best interests paramount. These challenges arise mainly from what I call "fiscal scarcity," the inadequacy of the funding necessary to make available to all needy patients the increasingly costly care now becoming standard throughout medicine. Fiscal scarcity, in turn, requires us to examine more carefully the legitimate competing claims of society, of payers, of other patients, and of other providers for the health care system's limited resources. Even more profoundly, it forces us to reconsider on a fundamental level what physicians and patients owe one another.

Moral problem-solving, in this context, will be both theoretical and practical. Theoretically, we will redefine physicians' fiduciary obligations as they arise, not in the context of the traditionally dyadic relationship, but as they emerge in the broader nexus of health care as a whole. And we will consider why it is morally imperative for patients to become more involved in medical decision-making and in its now-inevitable economic trade-offs. Practically, we will trace the specific implications that these redefined obligations have for clinical practice, and we can then explore the implications for patients as individuals and for national health policy. Overall, I hope it will become clear why, and how, the new economics of medicine provides an important opportunity not just to fashion the financial structure of health care in a more conscientious way, but to consider more carefully the basic values underlying that structure and the physician–patient relationship itself.

NOTES

1. Throughout this volume I will observe the somewhat old-fashioned but still correct custom of using the masculine pronoun in its gender-neutral

form to stand as the singular indefinite pronoun (see Shertzer, 1986, p. 20). To substitute plural pronouns such as "they" and "their" is incorrect; consistently using the feminine pronoun instead of the masculine is no less biased; and alternating between the two seems awkward and contrived.

2. Moore, 1989.

3. Throughout this volume I will mainly use the plural form of the first person pronoun. To me, an interested reader is not simply a passive recipient of the ideas on the pages, but an active participant in thinking through the issues discussed there. In deference to this joint undertaking of author and reader, then, I use "we" instead of "I."

4. Caplan, 1982; Caplan, 1983.

5. Brennan, 1987.

6. Gleick, 1987; Kass, 1990; Jonsen and Toulmin, 1988, pp. 21–46.

7. Gorovitz and MacIntyre, 1976.

8. For further discussion of uncertainty in medicine, see Gorovitz and MacIntyre, 1976; Katz, 1984; Eddy, 1984.

9. For an excellent further discussion of some challenging cases in moral diagnostics see Jackson and Youngner, 1979.

10. Morreim, 1986(a); see also Fleck, 1987, pp. 165–76.

11. Morreim, 1983(a); Morreim, 1990(b).

2

A Bit of History

We begin with the most salient feature of health care economics in the United States: over the past three decades the total cost of health care has risen exponentially, and those who pay for it are urgently trying to control their expenditures. This economic upheaval is triggering profound changes in the financing and delivery of health care and, thereby, is precipitating the moral challenges that are the focus of this volume. To understand how all this has come about, we must first examine the explosion of expenditures and its causes.

Health care in the United States was not always the costly item it is today. Before World War II, health care was largely delivered in homes by family members.[1] Physicians had relatively little to offer, save their conscientious attention and care. In 1929 health care represented only 3.5% of the Gross National Product (GNP), and even by 1950 this figure had risen to only 4.4%.[2] Since that time, however, annual health care expenditures in the U.S. have grown to over half a trillion dollars, more than 11% of the GNP.[3]

The problem, however, is not that this or that dollar or GNP figure is spent. Rather, it is the steady rise in expenditures and increasing proportion of total budgets that frightens those who pay for care.[4] Consider first the business community. When General Motors' Chairman Roger Smith announced in 1976 that GM was spending more on health benefits than on steel, the entire business community took note.[5] By 1984 GM's total tab for employee health benefits had grown to $2.35 billion, or $5000 per active worker.[6] That same year health benefits added $600 to the price of each Chrysler car.[7] By 1986 Chrysler's figure had risen to $700 per car, nearly $6000 per employee.[8] Though American auto workers in 1984 earned an hourly wage quite similar to that of their Japanese counterparts, the addition of fringe benefits—one of the largest of which is health care—rendered the difference substantial: $22/hr. in the U.S. versus $13.50/hr. in Japan.[9]

8

While business pays for nearly one-third of Americans' health care through their fringe benefits to employees, federal and state governments together pay for another 40%.[10] Federal Medicare outlays for the nation's elderly are projected to rise steadily. Although the exact numerical predictions change, it is generally agreed that not long after the turn of the century, Medicare will be the country's largest entitlement program, exceeding even Social Security, and that it will be massively in debt.[11] Meanwhile, Medicaid expenditures for the poor have often represented the largest and fastest growing part of states' budgets, in many cases rising faster than their revenues.[12] Overall, the United States spends more on health care than any other nation.[13] And yet this tremendous outlay does not necessarily bring us better health.[14]

How has this situation come about? There are a number of factors—economic, political, social, and normative—and we can survey them only briefly here. However, we can at least begin to understand not only why health care costs have escalated so aggressively but, more importantly, why this rise will probably continue and why those who pay for care are so determined to stop the trend.

SOURCES OF COST ESCALATION

Economic Factors

Shortly after World War II, the U.S. Government began to fund medical research, medical education, and hospital construction heavily, eager to improve citizens' lot after the lean years of depression and war. The National Institutes of Health became a showcase of science's best research, while the Hill–Burton program funded the construction of hospitals throughout the country.[15] With extensive government and private investment over the years, American medicine enjoyed a remarkable proliferation of high technology and advanced health care facilities and, with it, a shift from its formerly labor-intensive status to a capital- and technology-intensive enterprise.[16]

That shift has contributed substantially to cost escalation. While some observers believe that "little ticket" items such as lab tests and x-rays are especially responsible for technology-based cost increases,[17] others focus on the largest and costliest interventions. These include diagnostic technologies such as computerized tomography, magnetic resonance imaging, and positron emission tomography; the substitution of surgery for medical management of problems such as coronary artery disease; high-tech care of premature newborns; and intensive treatments of the critically ill.[18] This latter category has implications throughout health care, for nearly everyone can expect to die of something expensive.[19] In any given year, some 70% of Medicare funding is spent on only 9% of its beneficiaries, namely, those who are critically ill.[20] More broadly, we spend a large proportion of our health care dollars on people in their last year of life, up to 1% of the nation's total GNP.[21] Whether little ticket or big, these commentators warn that we will never curb overall health expenditures unless we are willing to constrain the development and utilization of our technology.[22]

Growing investment in research, technology, and construction has been accompanied by a proliferation of third-party funding to pay for its use. After the first Blue Cross plan was born in 1929 at Baylor University in Dallas, Texas, insurance soon became a standard work benefit enabling millions of middle-class Americans to enjoy the full benefits of improving medical technology. In 1965 those same benefits were extended by the Federal Government to cover the elderly and many of the poor.[23]

For its subscribers such insurance meant full access to the health care system. Reimbursement mechanisms not only compensated physicians and hospitals for all services rendered, but in effect encouraged them to provide any and all interventions that promised potential benefit. Typically, physicians and hospitals were retrospectively paid their usual, customary, and reasonable charges for each service rendered. Providers thereby had incentive to ensure that their fees were comfortably high and not subject to reduction; to perform as many services as possible; and to "unbundle" their care by describing each intervention as a number of separate services.[24] Further, because insurance companies would reimburse inpatient services more readily than outpatient, physicians tended to admit patients to the hospital for procedures or tests that might not otherwise be thought to require inpatient care. "The simplest fact of hospital operation . . . is the magnetism of an empty bed when payment for its use is assured."[25]

Essentially, the system was a "cost plus" pass-through arrangement in which providers who ordered care were usually paid what they asked of insurers, who in turn benefited as they sold more insurance and passed on higher premium costs to subscribers, mainly government and business.[26] The result was massive price inflation that, according to economist Kenneth Wing, may be the single most important factor in the overall rise of health care expenditures.[27]

Political Factors

These economic arrangements did not come about by chance. Public faith in science and technology, combined with a relentless popular demand for more and better health services,[28] ensured that government would be involved with health financing for the foreseeable future. Reciprocally, the enormous power of the medical profession following World War II ensured that, as both government and private insurance expanded, its terms would be substantially dictated by the medical profession, leaving them in control not only of their own professional services, but of health resources generally.[29]

The trend toward broad benefits under provider control was supported by a feeling in the U.S. and throughout the developed world that a person should not be forced to weigh costs and benefits at the time of illness—that individuals should not have to forgo needed care on account of cost at the time that care is rendered.[30] Thus both providers and patients were insulated from the economic consequences of their health care spending decisions. Indeed, many employees had first dollar coverage in their fringe benefit packages, exempting them entirely from any direct costs for health care.[31] Patients could freely demand "the best, no expenses spared," safe in the knowledge that insurance would cover the cost, while physicians could freely order every intervention of the slightest potential benefit.[32] In many cases, physicians did not even know the cost of the interventions they ordered.[33] Such insulation contributed to tremendous escalations in premium costs and in turn to the overall costs of care.

Social Factors

While these economic and political contributions to the cost of care are largely the products of human intervention, other factors are not. The U.S. population, for example, is growing older. The proportion of Americans over age 65 has risen steadily since the turn of the century, and those over 85 represent the fastest-growing age cohort. We could review a mind-numbing list of statistics,[34] but the bottom line requires no computer. With advanced age comes more illness, especially chronic diseases and disability.[35] And with higher numbers of aged come still more of the same. We already spend three and a half times more on the care of the elderly than on the rest of the population.[36] As the proportion of elderly rises, particularly that of the very old, there is little doubt that considerable increases in expenditures will be required to maintain current levels of care.

Expenditures must also rise if we intend to care for over thirty million Americans who lack medical insurance. Though Medicaid is intended to help such people, it covers not 65% of the poor as in the past, but only 38%, and in some states less than 25%.[37]

While governments and providers at all levels wrestle with this challenge,[38] an even larger, potentially even costlier, challenge looms: Acquired Immune Deficiency Syndrome (AIDS) and diseases related to the Human Immunodeficiency Virus (HIV). I will not even attempt to document here the number of patients with HIV or their associated medical costs. Estimates are difficult to formulate and they change regularly.[39] Even these tentative estimates do not begin to account for the less obvious costs of HIV-related diseases, such as lost productivity as young citizens are struck down. And with research successes come even higher costs. Drugs that ameliorate but do not cure AIDS ("half-way technologies," as Dr. Lewis Thomas has called them) may prolong useful life, but at the cost of further bouts of serious infection, a longer span of debilitation and dementia, or other unfortunate and costly complications.

Finally, Americans' litigiousness also has its cost. Physicians' fear of being sued may not always be based on a realistic appraisal of legal risks. Nevertheless, defensive medicine—typically characterized by the performance of otherwise-unnecessary interventions in order to minimize the chance of incurring or losing a lawsuit—may cost the nation up to $13 billion per year.[40] Malpractice tensions may be exacerbated as cost constraints pressure physicians to do less for patients, who in turn may notice with some anxiety or annoyance that their physicians are less willing than in earlier times to spare no expense in their care.

Normative Factors

The values we hold as individuals and as a society are a driving force in shaping our economic and political health care arrangements, and our collective response to such social factors as aging and AIDS. Deeply embedded in our attitudes and way of life, key values must be examined if we are to respond adequately to the new challenges of health care economics.

Some of our most powerful values concerning health and health care are in tension with each other. On the one hand most of us believe, as lovers of freedom, that individuals should be allowed to spend their money largely as they please, including to purchase the most exotic, state-of-the-art health care available.[41] But as a society we also are egalitarian enough to think that no one should be denied health care or other life-saving interventions simply because he cannot afford to pay.[42] The rule of rescue demands that "we throw a rope to the drowning, rush into burning buildings to snatch the entrapped, dispatch teams to search for the snowbound,"[43] and somehow find the money to fund the televised plea for organ transplant.

Between these values—the libertarian freedom of the affluent to buy all the health care they want and our egalitarian refusal to deny equivalent care to the poor—we find ourselves supposing that the poor are morally entitled to almost any health care that the wealthy can afford. The result is "an explosive chain reaction" of expenditures.[44]

In addition, we have tremendous faith in technology and in the power of science to cure what ails us.[45] The medical profession enthusiastically shares this value, embracing a technological imperative that favors intervention over inaction. If something can be done to find and fix the problem then it should be done, even at some risk of causing further harm.[46] Within the profession, physicians share an almost obsessive desire "to be complete," to think of every possibility, explore every option, eliminate every uncertainty.[47]

Beyond this, and perhaps most important, physicians have long insisted that their first loyalty must be to their patients. Patients' enormous vulnerability requires that they be able to trust not only that their physician is competent and skillful, but that he will pursue each patient's interests above his own or anyone else's.[48]

All these factors, then—economic, political, social, and normative—have fueled a virtually uncontrolled escalation of health care costs. Physicians and patients have pursued health care largely without regard to its price tag.

EARLY EFFORTS AT COST CONTAINMENT

Though health care costs have only recently become such an urgent national priority, serious efforts to limit spending in fact appeared much earlier. Both government and private insurance have always specified limits on eligibility and coverage, for example. Private insurance covers only its paid subscribers, while Federal Medicare money is reserved mainly for the elderly and Medicaid for the poor (with specific eligibility criteria varying considerably from state to state). Coverage for both private and government insurance has usually been restricted to medically necessary care, thereby excluding experimental interventions, screening tests, general checkups, and elective cosmetic surgery.[49] Insurers have always scrutinized the charges they are asked to pay, and in recent years have instituted closer scrutiny, more ready denials and delays of payment, and in some cases more restricted criteria of eligibility and coverage.[50]

These limitations did not prevent health care costs from rising faster than the rest of the economy, however, and as time went on more powerful measures were instituted. In 1971, for example, the Nixon administration applied a wage and price freeze that, even though generally lifted in 1973, was retained another year for health care and several other industries.[51] In 1972 Congress created Professional Standards Review Organizations (PSROs) to prevent excessive hospitalization and to limit other overutilization in the care of Medicare and Medicaid patients.[52] (Though PSROs did little to contain costs and were eventually dropped, they were basically reincarnated in 1982 as Peer Review Organizations [PROs], to monitor both utilization and quality of care for these same patients.[53]) In 1973 new legislation fostered health maintenance organizations, regarded as a promising vehicle to contain costs over the long run.[54] The next year Health Systems Agencies were created to restrain the proliferation and unnecessary duplication of costly technology, first by drawing up three-year health plans for each area of the country and second by reviewing proposals for new construction and large capital acquisition. All states were required to enact certificate-of-need legislation to ensure that only needed technologies and facilities were acquired within each region.[55]

These strategies generally failed, however, as highlighted in the mid-1970s by the "stagflation" that kept health care costs soaring amidst a sluggish economy. Under the Carter administration's threats of mandatory price controls, hospitals agreed in 1979 to restrain their revenues voluntarily. This program too had at most a short-lived, limited success.[56]

The largely failed strategy of government regulation was replaced by an increasing focus on competition within the health care industry,[57] beginning in 1982 with legislation to shift providers' incentives dramatically. The Tax Equity and Fiscal Reform Act (TEFRA) created Diagnostic Related Groups (DRGs), a system of prospective payment modeled after a plan that had been operating in New Jersey for several years. Instead of traditional cost-based retrospective reimbursement, hospitals caring for Medicare patients would now be paid according to a prospectively determined formula. With some adjustments for locality, case mix, and other factors, payment would now be based not on the number and nature of services performed for the patient, but primarily upon the patient's diagnosis as categorized by some 470 diagnostic groups. Because payment was now fixed, the hospital could pocket any money not used in the patient's care; reciprocally, however, it must make up the difference when care cost more than the reimbursement. Suddenly the old incentive to maximize services gave way to a new incentive to discharge patients rapidly and with as few interventions as possible.[58] Shortly after the initiation of DRGs, many states adopted similar prospective payment plans and an array of other devices to curb their own Medicaid costs.[59]

Prior to prospective payment and DRGs, cost containment efforts were relatively anemic and largely futile, as national health care expenditures continued to skyrocket.[60] The TEFRA legislation not only changed Federal payment incentives; it sparked the business community to launch its own far-ranging and powerful new cost containment initiatives. We will explore these in the next chapter. For now, we need to make only one point: for all their power, these new devices do not yet promise any serious and long-range reduction, or even adequate control, of health care costs. In fact, a whole collection of factors instead bodes continued escalation.

FUTURE ECONOMIC PRESSURES

Many cost containment devices result in one-time savings that temporarily diminish the baseline of medical expenditures without affecting the rate of growth. Hospital admissions and length of stay can be cut back, but only so far, and once clinical routines of care have had their "fat" trimmed, further reductions can compromise quality of care.[61] In other cases costs are not being reduced at all, but simply shifted to another setting. Tests formerly performed during a patient's hospital stay, for example, may now be performed as outpatient procedures before or after admission, without necessarily reducing the patient's length of stay. While the hospital may fare better by doing fewer things for the patient under its fixed reimbursement, or may even profit if those outpatient tests are done in a hospital-owned facility, third-party payers' costs in some cases may actually have gone up, not down.[62]

These theoretical projections are being borne out by data. Though the inflation rate in health care was considerably lower during the mid-1980s, that diminution was probably due mostly to a general marked decline in inflation. Even then, health care's cost escalation still vastly outpaced the general inflation rate and the GNP growth rate.[63] Since then, health care expenditures have once again far outpaced the general price index.

A number of factors conspire to keep those expenditures rising. We have already noted the expected impact of AIDS, aging, and indigency. Continuing technological developments, from positron emission tomography to laser holography, combined with our long-standing feeling of entitlement to "spare no expense" care, pressure the standard of care to rise ever higher at ever greater cost.[64]

Beyond this, entrepreneurial competition throughout the health care industry may be more likely to raise, not lower, overall expenditures, as least so long as health care financing is still largely open-ended. While competition can of course reduce the prices of individual products and services, its overall goal and probable effect will be to produce new types of services, greater numbers of services per patient, more (even if briefer) hospitalizations, more ancillary care, and a wider domain of services ranging from sports medicine to wellness to health education.[65] The purpose of entrepreneurial activity is, after all, to increase both the overall market and one's own share of that market. Expansion, not contraction, is the goal.

The increased costs of competition could be exacerbated by a projected surplus of physicians. According to a study by the Graduate Medical Education National Advisory Committee (GMENAC), we can anticipate a surplus of 140,000 physicians by the year 2000.[66] While the fees of individual physicians may come down, whether through competition or through changes in the ways in which physicians are paid,[67] overall health costs will quite likely rise if these predictions prove true. Each physician generates costs many times his own remuneration through the products, services, and hospitalization he orders for his patients. Since physicians control up to 80% of health care costs, a 20% increase in the number of physicians could generate up to 14% higher health care outlays overall.[68] In this sense, health care costs may be more attributable to the number of physicians than to the amount of illness in the society.[69]

The bottom line is simple and it is sobering. Cost containment is not succeeding.[70] However onerous physicians and patients may feel current economic constraints to be, they will surely become more stringent in the future. Payers' expenditures are sure to rise substantially if present trends continue, and those payers will not accede willingly to continued uncontrolled costs. American businesses' ability to compete in the international marketplace is threatened if they cannot control this substantial cost of production.[71] For their part, Federal and many state governments are wrestling with large deficits and have few ways to reduce them.[72] Many components of the Federal budget, for example, are off limits to deficit reduction. These include entitlement programs like Social Security, numerous fixed costs in national defense, and interest payments on the national debt.[73] With so little left from which to cut, health care programs stood as a prime target for cutbacks throughout the Reagan years and into the Bush administration. We can reasonably expect that for the foreseeable future, the looming national deficit will ensure the continued scrutiny of health care budgets.[74]

It is time, then, to examine how economics is changing the delivery of health care and, in particular, to describe the specific ways in which these changes bear on physicians. Only then will we be able to assess the moral challenges that the economic revolution in health care poses for physicians, now and in the future.

NOTES

1. Starr, 1982, p. 22.
2. Wing, 1986, p. 619.
3. Ginzberg, 1987, p. 1151.
4. Schwartz, 1987, p. 220.
5. Freedman, 1985, p. 580.
6. Demkovich, 1986, p. 59.
7. Thurow, 1985, p. 611.
8. Winslow, 1989.
9. Thurow, 1984, p. 1569. Other industries have fared similarly. See Butler and Haislmeyer, 1989, p. 17–18.
10. Ginzberg, 1987, p. 1153; Evans, 1986, p. 597.

11. Roper, 1988, p. 866; Board of Trustees Report, 1986; Hotchkiss, 1987, p. 947; Butler and Haislmaier, 1989, pp. 19, 70–75.

12. Wing, 1986, p. 657; Iglehart, 1983, p. 976; Butler and Haislmaier, 1989, pp. 91–97.

13. Schieber and Poullier, 1987, p. 108.

14. Shenkin, 1986; Lister 1986; Fuchs, 1986; Starr, 1982; Cluff, 1986; Avorn, 1986, pp. 211–13; Maloney and Reemtsma, 1985; Thurow, 1985.

15. Starr, 1982, pp. 333–51.

16. Reinhardt, in Relman and Reinhardt, 1986, p. 218.

17. Shenkin, 1986, p. 13.

18. Showstack, Stone, and Schroeder, 1985; Schwartz, 1987; Sheps, 1988; Council on Scientific Affairs, 1988.

19. Thurow, 1985, p. 611.

20. Ibid., p. 611–12.

21. Callahan, 1986, p. 252; Mitchell and Virts, 1986, p. 115.

22. Mitchell and Virts, 1986; W.B. Schwartz, 1987; Callahan, 1986; Wing, 1986; Callahan, 1990; Wennberg, 1990.

23. Starr, 1982, p. 295, 363–78; Butler and Haislmaier, 1989, pp. 6–17.

24. Starr, 1982, p. 385–86; Waters and Tierney, 1984, p. 1251; Light, 1983, p. 1316; Reinhardt, 1986.

25. Starr, 1982, p. 364, 385–86.

26. Thurow, 1984, p. 1570; Light, 1983, p. 1316; Thurow, 1985; Shenkin, 1986.

27. Wing, 1986, p. 610; Enthoven and Kronick, 1989(a). For an excellent discussion of the inflationary pressures created by the structure of health insurance in the U.S., see Butler and Haislmaier, 1989, pp. 6–33.

28. Ginzberg, 1990.

29. Starr, 1982; Light, 1983, p. 1316; Ginzberg, 1986, p. 757; Havighurst, 1986(c).

30. Aaron and Schwartz, 1984, p. 134.

31. Ginzberg, 1986, p. 758.

32. Thurow, 1984, p. 1570; Butler and Haislmaier, 1989, pp. 6–13.

33. Halper, 1987, p.161; Elkowitz, 1987, p.273; Tierney, Miller and McDonald, 1990, p. 1503.

34. Goldsmith, 1986, p. 3371; Avorn, 1986, p. 214; Schneider, 1989, p. 907; Mechanic, 1986, p. 165; Rowe, Grossman, Bond et al., 1987, p. 1425; Davis, 1986, p. 235; Evans, 1983(a), p. 2048–49.

35. Rogers, 1986, p. 212.

36. Wing, 1986, p. 622; Mechanic, 1986, p. 39.

37. McCarthy, 1988, p. 75; Freedman et al., 1988, p. 844; Wilensky, 1988.

38. Iglehart, 1983.

39. Scitovsky, 1988; Mueller, 1986, p. 251; Andrulis et al., 1987, p. 1344; Arno, 1987, p. 1376; Andrulis, Weslowski, and Gage, 1989.

40. Reynolds, Rizzo, and Gonzalez, 1987; Fine and Sunshine, 1986.

41. Thurow, 1984.

42. Ibid., 1984.

43. Jonsen, 1986, p. 174.

44. Thurow, 1984, p. 1570; Schramm, 1984; Reinhardt, 1986.

45. Starr, 1982, p. 335–47; Angell, 1985, p. 1205.

46. Aaron and Schwartz, 1984, p. 7; Callahan, 1986, p. 250; Scheff, 1963; Brett, 1981.

47. Gabbard, 1985; Hardison, 1979; Reuben, 1984; Lundberg, 1983; Kassirer, 1989; Morreim, 1990(b).

48. Fuchs, 1987, p. 1155; Fuchs, 1986, p. 315; Levinsky, 1984; Pellegrino, 1986; Hiatt, 1975; Veatch, 1986.

49. Starr, 1982, p. 290 ff.

50. Iglehart, 1987(a), p. 642.

51. Starr, 1982, p. 399.

52. Ginzberg, 1987, p. 1151; Dans, Weiner, and Otter, 1985,p. 1131.

53. Shenkin, 1986, p. 69.

54. Starr, 1982, p. 400; Shenkin, 1986, p. 75.

55. Aaron and Schwartz, 1984, pp. 4–5; Starr, 1982, pp. 398, 402.

56. Aaron and Schwartz, 1984, p. 4; Fuchs, 1987, p. 1154; Starr, 1982, p. 414.

57. Blendon, 1986, p. 133; Starr, 1982, p. 418–19; Reinhardt, 1986; Ginzberg, 1986, p. 759; McDowell, 1989, p. 63–64, 71–72; Hyman and Williamson, 1988, pp. 1133, 1136, 1188; Blumstein and Sloan, 1981; Butler and Haislmaier, 1989, pp. 19–25.

58. Dans, Weiner, and Otter, 1985, p. 1131 ff.; Iglehart, 1985(a), p. 133; Shenkin, 1986, p. 69.

59. Kapp, 1984, p. 246.

60. Starr, 1982; Schwartz, 1981; Wing, 1986, p. 619; Sapolsky, 1986; Butler and Haislmaier, 1989, pp. 17–25.

61. Ginzberg, 1987, p. 1152–53; Schwartz, 1987, pp. 221–22; Ginzberg, 1983; Spivey, 1984, p. 985.

62. Reinhardt, 1986; Mitchell and Virts, 1986, p. 112.

63. Iglehart, 1987(a), p. 640.

64. Schwartz, 1987, p. 222; Schramm, 1984; Callahan, 1990.

65. Mechanic, 1986, p. 62; Ginzberg, 1987, p. 1153; Robinson and Luft, 1987; Robinson, Garnick and McPhee, 1987; Robinson et al., 1988.

66. Salmon, 1987.

67. Lee et al., 1989; Board of Trustees Report, 1989; Hsiao, Braun, Dunn, et al., 1988; Hsiao et al., 1987; U.S. Congress, 1989, p. H–9354 ff.

68. Ginzberg, 1987, p. 1152.

69. Fuchs, 1986, p. 275; Mechanic, 1986, p. 36; Maloney and Reemtsma, 1985, p. 1713; Evans, 1986. Some observers have questioned the predicted surplus of physicians. See Schwartz, Sloan, and Mendelson, 1988; Schloss, 1988.

70. Ginzberg, 1987; Evans, 1986; Altman and Rodwin, 1988; Sapolsky, 1986.

71. Thurow, 1985; Freedman, 1985; Thurow, 1984; Fuchs, 1987, p. 1155; Winslow, 1989. Disagreeing: Reinhardt, in Relman and Reinhardt, 1986, p. 210; Reinhardt, 1989.

72. Blendon et al., 1986.

73. Iglehart, 1987(a), p. 639; Iglehart, 1985(b), p. 525.

74. For a useful discussion arguing that our system of health care financing is structurally flawed and inherently assured to produce both continued cost escalation and restricted access, see Butler and Haislmaier, 1989.

3

Economic Forces, Clinical Constraints

BROAD ECONOMIC FORCES

To understand just what challenges physicians face as a result of the economic overhaul of health care, we need first to note some fundamental features of the U.S. health care system. In its broadest outline, that system is more or less a free market. Much of its financing is private, as are most of its providers. Within certain regulatory parameters, citizens have free opportunity to become providers (sellers), offering a diversity of health care services and facilities ranging from major hospitals to sports and wellness clinics. This is unlike systems in which a government, acting as sole overall provider, determines how many of which facilities and services will be established to serve which citizens. The free-market system also features a wide variety of purchasers (buyers), in contrast to those systems in which government is sole purchaser on behalf of all eligible citizens. This free-market approach is based on the belief that if individuals are free to buy and sell goods based on their own preferences, it will be possible most efficiently to satisfy citizens' wants and needs, to improve quality of care with innovative services and products, and to keep prices down through vigorous competition.[1]

Admittedly, the U.S. health care system hardly fits perfectly the paradigm of free-market capitalism. As many economists have noted, important conditions of true markets are absent or even unattainable in the health care setting. The consumer of care—the patient—often is not sufficiently informed to decide his own preferences unless he relies heavily on the knowledge and advice of his physician.[2] Partly because of this consumer information problem, the health care market is quite heavily regulated. Key providers such as physicians must be licensed and bear clear responsibilities to act as fiduciaries in their patients' best interests. Key products such as drugs and medical devices require detailed approval procedures before they can be marketed and a physician's prescription before they can be purchased.

In addition, the health care market features an odd split between those who make the spending decisions (namely, patients in consultation with their physicians) and those who in most cases actually pay for those spending decisions (namely, the third-party payers such as insurance companies, business corporations, or government). In this sense, the term "purchaser" is systematically ambiguous: we could be referring either to patients or to payers. As we have already noted, this split is not accidental. Health insurance historically has been deliberately structured to insulate patients from worrying about costs at the time of illness, an arrangement that is not only highly inflationary, but also market-distorting.[3]

Finally, physicians' role is also ambiguous. While clearly they are providers selling their professional services, in an important sense they are also purchasers, since physicians exercise enormous power over patients' access to medical interventions and over their decisions about what medical care to buy. Indeed, one of the most important facts about health care economics is that physicians quite literally spend other people's money and distribute other people's property to their patients. This duality poses powerful moral challenges, as we will see throughout this volume.

Our aim here is neither to praise nor to criticize the American (quasi)free market system or any other approach to health care financing and distribution. Rather, the point is only that, however distant from the Adam Smith paradigm, the U.S. health care system does have certain central features of free markets. There are sellers, who aim to boost profits by selling as much product as possible while keeping their costs of production as low as possible. And there are buyers, who aim to secure the best value per dollar in the products and services they buy, and to spend as few dollars on those purchases as possible. In health care, this translates into myriad providers, such as hospitals and freestanding imaging centers, vigorously marketing their services to gain greater market shares. Reciprocally, we see them cutting their costs of operation by enhancing efficiency and eliminating unprofitable services or unprofitable patients. Purchasers, in like manner, are pursuing value for their dollars by requiring providers to demonstrate empirically that their medical interventions actually make a difference in health outcomes.[4] And like the providers, they are vigorously trying to hold down their costs.

Interestingly, at least three of these four basic forces of the U.S. health care system can be found in virtually any system. Although not all systems feature providers seeking profits, providers everywhere need to be efficient, stretching their resources as far as possible. And purchasers, including governments, likewise need to stretch their resources, buying quality care while conserving dollars, rubles, yen, pounds, or kroner. Recent years have witnessed strains in health care systems around the world, as all nations address the resource problems posed by costly new medical technology, national deficits, competing national priorities, and rising public expectations.[5]

We turn, then, to see more specifically how these broad forces affect those who purchase and provide health care and, ultimately, how they impinge upon physicians in clinical decision-making.

INSTITUTIONAL PAYERS AND PROVIDERS

In order to understand the ways in which economic changes in health care challenge physicians and their traditional obligations to patients, we must pay special attention to what I will call the "economic agents" of health care. These are especially the institutional payers and providers who immediately own or pay for the use of the medical and monetary resources of care. This is not to deny, of course, that individual physicians are providers, or that individual patients are also payers. Patients do, after all, pay some medical bills out of their own pockets and, in an ultimate sense, are the ones who finance the institutional payers and providers through their premiums and their patronage. We will examine patients' economic role more closely in later chapters. For now, however, we must recognize that patients' direct financial involvement in health care is ordinarily very limited. Few patients pay more than a small portion of their actual medical bills, and even those who hold stock in publicly traded health care corporations can rarely claim more than the most marginal status as an owner of health care resources. Neither, usually, does the physician own many of the technologies that he delivers to patients, whether hospital beds or computerized tomography scans, although that situation has begun to change.[6]

If we wish to understand how changes in medical economics will affect physicians and patients, therefore, we need to begin by recognizing that the economic pressures affecting clinical decision-making are created primarily by the economic agents who directly own or control the resources of care. These economic agents include institutional purchasers—both private and governmental third-party payers, who furnish most of the fiscal resources of health care—and institutional providers, who provide the physical resources of care, ranging from hospital beds and the nurses who staff them, to sophisticated technologies such as magnetic resonance imagers, to the smaller commodities of care such as bedpans and pain pills. We will look first at economic agents' role in the health care system. Following that, we will see that although these agents differ substantially in form and function, they all tend to use the same basic devices for influencing physicians' clinical decisions about the use of their medical and monetary resources.

Institutional Payers

Three kinds of institutional payers are particularly prominent: private insurers, governments, and business corporations. Private insurance companies are the health care financiers with which many people are most familiar. They have existed far longer than government insurance programs—1929 versus 1965, respectively—and they commonly stand as the fiscal intermediaries through which employers provide workers' health care benefits. Even people with government insurance may also subscribe to private plans; for instance, elderly citizens purchase "Medi-Gap" plans to cover the copayments and deductibles left by Medicare insurance.

For many years, private insurers acted essentially as a pass-through system for the burgeoning costs of health care. Unlike other forms of insurance that protect against improbable, fixed-cost losses such as the burning of a house, health care expenses are as open-ended as health needs and as expansive as our ever-growing technology.[7] Until recently, insurers actually benefited from the rising costs of health care, because higher health care costs meant larger premiums and thereby larger profits.[8] However, as businesses and individual subscribers now refuse to accede to skyrocketing annual premium increases, insurance companies have developed an array of devices to curb their reimbursement outlays. We will examine them below.

Government, whether Federal or state, has basically two ways in which to contain its health care costs: regulation and incentives. In regulation, a government makes explicit rules to limit how much of its (and sometimes others') money is spent to do what for whom. As we have seen, Medicare and Medicaid have always restricted eligibility—respectively, to the elderly and those with particular disabilities such as end-stage renal disease, and to the poor. And they have always limited coverage, favoring medically necessary care over routine care, explicitly rejecting experimental interventions and clearly elective procedures. In recent years, limits on eligibility and coverage have become increasingly stringent.[9]

Governments also can alter their manner and rates of reimbursement. The shift to DRGs represented a major change in the way in which hospitals were paid for Medicare patients. National and state governments are also experimenting with capitated approaches, in which providers or financial intermediaries are given a single sum of money to care for each patient for the entire year. And physicians' reimbursement—which under Medicare Part B represents the nation's fourth largest domestic Federal expense[10]—is now based on a relative value scale.[11]

Regulation can affect not just persons and payments, but the facilities and daily details of care as well. We have already noted that Health Systems Agencies and Certificate of Need programs were established to restrain unnecessary proliferation of costly technologies and capital construction. Professional Standards Review Organizations (PSROs) in the 1970s and their 1980s incarnation, the Peer Review Organizations (PROs), tried to require physicians to develop more efficient standards of care.[12] And in some cases regulation has meant rationing policies, as for example through explicit criteria governing which patients will be eligible for an organ transplant or an artificial heart.[13]

Though regulation strategies have had their successes[14] and failures,[15] recent government efforts have focused more on incentives and on encouraging competition in the private sector.[16] In the state of California, for example, providers who wish to care for Medi-Cal (California's Medicaid) patients must compete with other providers to offer the state the most attractive package of fees and services. Successful applicants are then assured a substantial volume of these patients, who are required to secure their care from designated providers.[17] At the Federal level, hospitals wishing to perform government-reimbursed heart transplants must demonstrate that they will be effective and efficient providers. Since the applicable criteria include the institution's volume of transplants, competition is implicit.[18]

Ultimately the relationship between government policies (whether regulatory or competitive) and clinical decisions is fairly simple: it is easier to provide reimbursed care for well-insured patients, and it is more difficult to offer interventions that will not be reimbursed or are in limited supply or to care for patients who are not insured.

Though government was the prime mover of cost containment during the early 1980s, the business community is rapidly taking the lead.[19] Initially their strategies focused on increasing employees' responsibility for health and health care, and on reducing inpatient delivery of care. Employees' increased responsibility took several forms. Foremost, they were required to pay higher coinsurance, copayments, and deductibles. When both common sense and careful studies indicated that health care utilization falls as out-of-pocket expenses increase,[20] employers rapidly began to eliminate the first-dollar coverage that had long insulated workers from considering whether a proposed medical intervention was worth its cost.[21]

Beyond this, firms have encouraged employees to adopt healthier lifestyles by instituting on-the-job wellness education, fitness programs, and even elaborate exercise facilities. Some corporations have offered financial incentives to shed pounds, discard cigarettes, buckle seat belts, and reduce drinking habits,[22] while others outright forbid or substantially restrict their employees' use of tobacco or other unhealthy substances.

Businesses have reduced hospitalization, which accounts for some 40% of total health care expenditures, in a variety of ways. Benefit packages have been altered to encourage or require second opinions on selected surgeries; to reimburse outpatient surgeries and diagnostic procedures more attractively than inpatient treatment; to cover home nursing care and extended care facilities; to exclude or severely restrict nonemergency weekend admissions; to require prospective authorization and concurrent length-of-stay review for all hospital admissions; and to subject hospital bills retrospectively to ever closer audit.[23]

In addition to these early attempts to tinker with specific benefits and expenditures, corporations are now attempting to overhaul quite fundamentally their systems of financing and delivering workers' health care.[24] They are not only embracing alternative delivery systems such as Health Maintenance Organizations (HMOs) and Preferred Provider Organizations (PPOs), but are inducing competition among all providers by offering their employees choices.[25] Thus, in 1985 General Motors initiated its Informed Choice Plan, offering workers an HMO, a PPO, and a traditional fee-for-service package equipped with careful utilization controls.[26] Not only do these designated providers have to compete with each other for workers' allegiance, they must constantly compete with other HMOs and PPOs to retain their place as designated providers. They must offer the best service package at the best price. In other cases, businesses may actually require workers to enroll in an HMO or other designated plan, at least for an initial trial period.[27]

One of the greatest changes is a massive shift away from purchasing health benefits through such fiscal intermediaries as insurance companies, toward self-insurance in which the corporation directly assumes full responsibility for employees' health care. As the corporation directly provides or contracts for health care, it is able more precisely to monitor its costs and to reap the rewards of prudent management.[28]

A still bigger change, only recently, is the emergence of major corporations' support for the concept of national health insurance. Discouraged with failures to contain their health care costs and now doubtful that such efforts will ever succeed, some corporations argue that no real control will be achieved until there is a coherent national health care system.[29] As the impetus is relatively new, its effects remain to be seen. But in combination with some physician groups and others advocating the same conclusion,[30] a further and even more radical restructuring of the U.S. health care economy is not beyond the realm of possibility.

Institutional Providers

If the institutional purchasers of care are looking to contain their costs and secure value for their dollars, the institutional providers are looking to survive and produce a profit (or a surplus, in the case of non-profit providers), while vigorously containing their own costs. Hospitals are undoubtedly the most familiar institutional providers. Because hospitals, not physicians, are the direct targets of such cost containment schemes as the Medicare DRG plan, they have been forced to examine their operations and facilities carefully. Competitive hospitals now offer a wide variety of new services to boost their revenues, from acquiring the latest medical technologies; to instituting helicopter transport services, free-standing ambulatory satellite clinics, inpatient psychiatric units, and home health care agencies; to establishing such non-health-care businesses as parking garages, real estate firms, and gourmet restaurants. Cost containment reciprocally has prompted many hospitals to reduce staff, eliminate unprofitable services, and even to eliminate unprofitable patients by transferring them to public hospitals or discharging them quickly to nursing homes.[31] Multihospital corporations have also become prominent, though early predictions that they would dominate the entire health care industry later faded.[32]

Hospitals are not the only provider-institutions. HMOs, which function doubly as providers and insurers, have established a solid foothold in the health care market. HMOs were initially inspired by the observation that the traditional fee-for-service reimbursement encouraged overutilization. If insurers would pay for procedures in the hospital but not outside, the physician would naturally admit the patient. If insurers paid a separate fee for each service, the incentive was to perform more procedures. And as preventive care was not covered, illnesses might be ignored until they were more serious and more expensive. Under radically different economic arrangements, so the reasoning went, physicians might be inspired to focus more on health and prevention, and to provide only necessary care in the least intensive setting. Thus the HMO was conceived, in which patients pay a single, usually annual, fee for all health services. Many HMOs provide their own hospitals and outpatient facilities, hire their own medical and ancillary staffs, and thus constitute completely self-contained providers. Other HMOs, while still billing patients a single sum per year, nevertheless contract with existing facilities and independently practicing physicians for their services. This independent practice association (IPA), a variant of the HMO, gained popularity because of its lower start-up costs and its greater variety of physicians from which patients may choose. Unlike the salaried staff physicians of the staff-model HMOs, IPA physicians are more likely to be paid fee-for-service, or a capitated annual fee for each of their enrolled patients.[33]

The independent practice corporation (IPC) is a still newer genre of the HMO. Instead of offering their services directly to patients, IPC physicians incorporate to offer their services to insurance companies. The insurer pays a fixed cost, while participating physicians receive their payment according to the corporation's chosen formula. Chief among its advantages, advocates say, is the fact that the physicians are in control not only of patient care, but also of the economic success of the corporation. Because they therefore undertake their own utilization review and other cost containment procedures, the physicians are better able to retain their clinical authority in patient care with less outside interference.[34]

A PPO, in contrast, is not a direct provider of care, but rather a kind of broker between physicians and/or hospitals on the one hand, and insurance companies, businesses, or other purchasers on the other. That broker may be a separate agency, or may simply be the collection of providers. In either case, providers offer their services to purchasers at negotiated, usually reduced, rates. Purchasers assure these providers a steady volume of patients by giving patients strong financial incentives to select the preferred providers for their care. For example, an insurance company might reimburse the patient 90% for care from a preferred hospital or physician, but only 70% for care obtained outside the approved panel. In addition to negotiating reduced fees, purchasers typically institute utilization controls and other economic restraints, to be discussed below.[35]

In another variation, managed fee-for-service is available in a variety of forms. This approach features traditional fee-for-service care, but incorporates assorted controls and utilization review.[36]

Finally, in response to the Federal Government's invitation to "go ye and compete," a wide variety of other providers is emerging, from freestanding ambulatory clinics, surgical facilities, and diagnostic imaging centers to laboratories, home health agencies, physical therapy services, and independent dietetic businesses.

In this keenly competitive environment where marketing is virtually as important as medicine, institutional providers need to enlist the close cooperation of physicians. Although hospitals, HMOs, PPOs, and clinics can determine what technologies they will acquire and what staff they will hire, the fact remains that physicians control up to 80% of actual health care spending through their decisions about what products and services to offer to which patients, and whom to hospitalize for how long, at what level of nursing care.[37] Therefore, institutional providers and payers must translate their own economic pressures into clinical constraints upon physicians.

CLINICAL CONSTRAINTS

The devices by which institutional providers and payers inspire physicians to contain costs or boost revenues are numerous and varied, and it is important to recognize that they are imposed by both payers and providers, each group working toward its own respective goals. Broadly, we may distinguish between *controls* and *incentives*. With controls, an outside party literally dictates the physician's decision or substantially restricts his options. Incentives, on the other hand, leave the physician clinically free to offer the patient whichever interventions he wishes, but pose consequences to influence that decision. Financial rewards or penalties, professional privileges, or peer esteem may all be interposed between the physician and his decision. Let us inventory, then, the ways in which institutional providers and payers influence clinical decisions.

Direct Controls

Institutional payers and providers have devised many ways in which to restrict physicians' options or direct their decisions. A hospital-based laboratory, for example, might refuse to honor more than a specified number of "stat" (immediate service) orders per day from any one physician, or may restrict stat orders to emergency or acute care units.[38] An HMO or a hospital's pharmacy formulary may decline to stock certain costly drugs, or may automatically substitute generic for brand-name medications.[39] In other cases the pharmacy may routinely make "therapeutic substitutions" of a chemically different compound that is believed to have the same effect as the prescribed drug.[40] Or the physician may be required to follow a step care protocol requiring that he try a drug from one class before ordering one from any higher class.[41]

A hospital or its radiology department might refuse to carry new types of low-osmolar or nonionic contrast dyes, which cause less morbidity and mortality but at far higher cost than more traditional contrast media. Or they might purchase these costly dyes but reserve them only for high-risk patients—perhaps defining high-risk in some very narrow way.[42] Similarly, a primary care physician may be forbidden to order the costliest interventions without the approval of an administrator or of a consultant in the relevant field.[43] In other cases, major decisions such as selection of organ transplant recipients may be left in the hands of committees or a collectively constructed formula.[44]

Such direct controls over medical decisions are of limited use, however. As we will see in the next chapter, it is undesirable if not impossible to dictate too intimately the daily details of medical care.[45] Therefore, physicians are subjected to other influences.

Education

The earliest and surely most benign effort at cost containment was simply to educate physicians about the economic implications of their spending decisions, in the Platonic hope that with knowledge would come virtue. Insulated as they and their patients were from the costs of care, many physicians often did not even know the costs of the interventions they ordered.[46] Hospitals and other institutional providers attempted to remedy this problem by posting price lists of various procedures and medications in prominent places, and also by conducting seminars, chart audits, and other in-house educational efforts to urge physicians to consider not just the monetary costs, but the real medical value of their care. Such approaches, unfortunately, yielded little savings.[47]

This is not to say that they are irredeemably useless. Some observers have argued, for example, that such educational efforts have foundered not on any intrinsic lack of worth, but on inadequate teaching techniques. On one view, we might take a lesson from pharmaceutical representatives, who use a variety of powerful educational approaches to elicit the desired (purchasing) behavior. Perhaps those same techniques, properly applied, could substantially improve cost effectiveness in clinical decision making.[48]

A newer sort of education may also be effective. Many hospitals and even insurers and business firms are busy compiling computer profiles of individual physicians, comparing each one's practice patterns and spending habits with those of his colleagues. High-spending physicians might be inspired into more thrifty routines of care as such tallies are shared with clinicians or even openly distributed at staff meetings.[49] Reciprocally, some profit-seeking firms may use the same collegial comparisons to encourage staff physicians to perform higher volumes of lucrative procedures.[50]

Peer Pressure and Selective Recruiting

The embarrassment that may accompany open revelation of one's spending patterns identifies a potent economic tool: peer pressure. Physicians, perhaps more than any other profession, rely on one another not merely for collegiality and general advancement of the profession, but to construct collectively the informal routines by which physicians manage the myriad details and uncertainties so unavoidable in medicine.[51] Peer guidance is one of the predominant ways by which physicians learn medicine, and peer approval is a key index of one's satisfactory performance within the profession.[52] Even our legal system recognizes this power of peerage as it permits physicians, almost alone among professionals, to set their own legal standards of care.[53]

It should come as no surprise, then, that many HMOs recruit physicians carefully to ensure that they practice conservative medicine, or that hospitals increasingly consider physicians' economic performance in their credentialing process.[54] The more institutional providers can assemble staffs of like-minded conservative practitioners, the easier it becomes to sway higher-spending physicians to adopt the wider group's norms.

Utilization Review

Whatever the value of education and peer pressure, far more stringent economic devices have been installed throughout the health care industry. One of these, utilization review, involves outside scrutiny of physicians' medical decisions. It comes in three basic forms: retrospective, prospective, and concurrent.

Retrospective review, the oldest, refers to insurance companies' or other payers' practice of looking carefully at the bills they are asked to pay, and electing in some instances to deny or reduce reimbursement on such grounds as lack of medical necessity, inadequate documentation of services, or excessive charges.[55] Though patients may be disappointed to learn after-the-fact that they must pay personally for care they thought would be covered, retrospective review has been upheld in common law as a useful and appropriate procedure.[56]

Prospective review, in contrast, requires that physicians secure prior approval of nonemergency hospitalization or of specified diagnostic studies, surgeries, and other costly interventions.[57] In like manner, concurrent review examines ongoing care to ascertain whether it is (still) medically necessary. Emergency admissions are thus subjected to next-day scrutiny, hospitalized patients' lengths of stay are questioned, discharge planning is facilitated, and ongoing care is challenged.[58] The HMO may inquire whether the child admitted with acute asthma really needs to stay longer than two days, or the insurance company's "patient advocate" may ask a physician whether Mrs. Jones still has her intravenous line, how soon she will be ready for discharge, and whether perhaps she can leave sooner if home nursing care is provided.

All three types of utilization review represent an interesting mix of controls and incentives. Technically, utilization review personnel do not control medical decisions at all. They control reimbursement. Yet clearly there is an intimate connection between money and health choices in the high-cost world of health care. A denial of funding, although not strictly determinative, represents a powerful constraint on care.[59]

Within this overall framework, an especially fast-growing structure for utilization review is the *case management system.* Actually, the term represents two quite different devices. In its older sense, case management refers to the social work concept of helping the client to find his way through a confusing morass of programs and bureaucracies. It means tailoring the individual person's assistance to his particular needs.[60]

In medicine this concept is applied to patients with especially difficult or unusual needs. Where the parents of a severely handicapped child are willing to care for their child at home but cannot afford the necessary equipment and nursing assistance because their insurance will only cover inpatient care, a case manager may seek some happy resolution wherein parents receive what they need to care for him at home while the insurance company saves substantially over the costs of inpatient care.[61]

A second, quite different, sort of case management refers to the primary care "gatekeeper" system employed by many HMOs and other highly structured delivery systems.[62] Under this approach the patient must select one primary care physician who not only coordinates, but controls his access to the entire health care system. That physician must approve all hospitalization, special consults, ancillary services, and other health interventions.[63]

Incentives

Merely to establish a physician as gatekeeper is unlikely of itself to lead to reduced use of services. If physicians believe it is their moral duty to provide patients with every intervention of even the most "infinitesimal benefit,"[64] or if they fear a legal risk from doing less than everything for the patient, then they are unlikely to hold back in their delivery of care.

Aware of these and other pressures on physicians to maximize interventions, virtually all institutional providers and payers of

health care have initiated financial and professional incentives—
"sticks and carrots"—that give the physician a personal, vested interest in economizing on care. A hospital administrator may send ominous letters of warning to physicians whose patients overspend their
welcome, or may limit physicians' access to costly technologies.[65] The
threat of losing hospital staff privileges or being dropped from an
HMO or PPO provider panel are more potent yet.[66]

More commonly, incentives are financial. They come in a stagger-
ing array of shapes and sizes, which we can only begin to appreciate
through some specific examples.

Hospitals, for example, employ assorted financial incentives. In
some cases a hospital will lease to the physician inexpensive office
space and equipment, or provide record keeping and billing services,
even malpractice insurance, with the implicit understanding that the
physician's admission and inpatient practices will be sufficiently
lucrative to the hospital.[67] In other cases a hospital may share its profits with cost-conscious physicians.[68] One investor-owned hospital
company, for example, "proposed sharing operating room revenues
with surgeons who use the facility, and another has proposed a profit-
sharing plan based on splitting surplus revenues, if any, derived"
under DRGs from the care of Medicare patients.[69] Subsequently, Congress outlawed the most offensive of such provisions.[70]

Hospitals may also offer global financial incentives by entering
into corporate joint ventures with physicians, in which both share
directly in the economic risks and profits of the hospital.[71]

Insurance companies employ their own incentives. The oldest
and probably most effective is their prerogative to deny reimbursement. With ever closer utilization review, insurance companies can
affect physicians' and hospitals' pocketbooks powerfully by their
refusals to pay. This incentive is nearly as potent when it is the patient
who is denied reimbursement, for his anger bodes not only lost business in the future, but in some cases the ominous threat of litigation.

Some insurance companies have gone beyond this to offer physicians direct bonuses for cost-conscious care. In 1984 Blue Cross/Blue
Shield of Kansas, for example, required tonsillectomies and some
sixty other elective surgical procedures to be performed on an outpatient basis, barring special circumstances, and in general paid physicians an extra $50–$100 to keep patients out of the hospital.[72]
Similarly, Blue Cross/Blue Shield of North Carolina began in 1981 to
pay surgeons bonuses of up to 25% to perform some eighty-eight

designated procedures outside the hospital, while Blue Shield of Massachusetts would pay an obstetrician more if his patient's length of stay after delivery was shorter than average. In all these cases the insurance company specified that the more economical care must still comport with accepted standards.[73] Still, the physician received cash payments to reduce the intensity of care.

Just as there are incentives to contain costs, incentives can also boost revenues. A walk-in clinic, for example, might give monthly bonus awards to those staff physicians generating the best sales figures[74] or may pay its physician-employees on the basis of the gross revenue they generate.[75]

HMOs' financial incentives have probably been most carefully studied.[76] Because most HMOs rely on the gatekeeper system, primary care physicians are their primary target. And because an HMO must operate within the fixed annual budget of patients' capitation payments, incentives appear primarily as a sharing of leftover premium dollars. That is, the more frugally the primary care physicians use hospitals, tests, and consultants, the more money is left at the end of the year. To encourage such frugality, most HMOs therefore withhold portions of the primary physician's income, to be returned or not at the end of the year according to the HMO's financial condition.[77]

Beyond this generic description, however, gatekeeper incentive arrangements vary tremendously. The amount withheld from the physician's fees, salary, or capitation payment may range from 11% to 30% or more, with the higher figures found in for-profit HMOs.[78] Formulae withholding less than 11% have been found to be inadequate as an incentive.[79]

Year-end surpluses may be distributed according to a number of formulae. All physicians might receive the same fixed percentage or fixed dollar amount, or each physician may be rewarded according to his personal productivity and frugality, as measured by his total number of patient visits, the total number of patients in his panel, total number of hospital days consumed by his patients, or the like. In some cases the physician may also profit as an investor in the HMO.[80]

Reciprocally, some 30% of HMOs place physicians at risk beyond the amount withheld. If the HMO does poorly during the year, physicians may have to pay back some of their nonwithheld income, incur liens on future earnings, or receive reduced capitation or a stiffer withholding percentage the next year.[81] The impact of such incentives on a physician's income[82] and on his behavior[83] can be substantial.

HMOs do not restrict their incentives to such withholding arrangements. Some also attach bonuses and penalties to specific patient care decisions. If a gatekeeper physician refers his patient to an emergency room for what is later judged by the HMO to have been not an emergency, he may be forced to pay the ER bill out of his own pocket.[84] One San Antonio HMO was reported to pay its obstetricians $600 for delivering a patient who stays in the hospital for three days; if she is gone within 24 hours his fee jumps to $1025.[85] Analogously, a Maryland HMO reportedly decided to curb the use of sonograms, fetal monitoring, and non-stress tests for pregnant women. Under their plan, the previous physician fee of $1200 per delivery (with a 30% withhold) was raised to $1700 for routine vaginal delivery and $2100 for cesarean delivery (with no withhold). However, the costs of these three tests would now be directly deducted from the physician's fee.[86] In a very real sense, the physician in this plan was required to pay for the patient's tests out of his own pocket. In the same vein, about 40% of HMOs take the costs of outpatient laboratory tests directly out of the fund that provides gatekeeper physicians' own salaries, fees, or capitation payments.[87] In all these arrangements, the physician earns more by doing less.

Finally, HMOs may also exert noneconomic incentives. Where the physician must spend unwieldy amounts of time in telephone haggling and in writing documentations in order to secure authorizations for specific medical interventions or consultant referrals, his threshold for determining which care is medically necessary may become considerably more conservative.[88]

Aside from the many incentives placed upon physicians by institutional payers and providers, some physicians actively place themselves under incentives as they become owners or major investors in free-standing or in-office facilities to which they may then refer their own patients. Such investments, particularly those in free-standing facilities, are a relatively recent phenomenon. For one thing, reimbursement policies that have changed to favor outpatient over inpatient care have created a market for outpatient facilities, such as ambulatory surgery and diagnostic centers, and home nursing and other service agencies. For another, the development of new technologies, such as magnetic resonance imaging and lithotripsy, creates a further demand for new facilities. Finally, as cost containment efforts become increasingly focused on physicians' incomes, physicians have still more reason to be interested in outside investments.[89]

These investments, obviously, can create incentives for physicians as they themselves become institutional providers. The more patients who utilize one's facility, the more it will flourish. Where the physician can refer his own patients to it, he has some incentive to prescribe that service for as many patients as possible, and to refer them to his own rather than to some alternative facility. Like the physician who is an employee in a for-profit firm, his incentive is to do more interventions, rather than to do fewer, wherever it is likely that the patient will pay his bills. Reciprocally, he also has the institutional providers' incentive to keep down his costs of operation by being frugal in his acquisitions of materials and supplies and in staff hiring practices.

Competition

A final source of substantial economic pressure comes from the physician's own colleagues, and in particular from their burgeoning numbers.[90] In a time of tightening health dollars and a relatively stable total population, this can mean fewer patients and less money per physician,[91] particularly in some areas of the country. Where there is such a surplus, individual physicians will compete with each other for patients, specialists will fight "turf battles" for jurisdiction over professional practices, referral patterns may be revised dramatically, and groups of physicians will compete with hospitals and corporations for the allegiance of patients.[92] Young physicians, often emerging from medical school with heavy debts,[93] may be increasingly tempted to opt for the economic security of the large corporation or HMO. Physician surplus and competition, in other words, can drive many physicians right into those very kinds of practice with the most highly structured cost containment, and which may thereby most restrict their professional freedom and judgment.

SUMMARY

We may conclude this survey of global and clinical economic pressures with a few general observations. First, we can identify some basic parameters along which cost constraints vary. They vary according to the extent to which they literally control the physician's decisions or leave him free to follow his own professional judgment; the size and type of incentive, whether monetary or professional sticks or carrots; and the directness of the incentive's connection with individual patient care decisions. As we will see later, these parameters can be morally important.

Second, the impetus to restrain health care is not necessarily bad. There are many ways in which the medical profession can reduce quantity of care without impairing quality. Further, there remain many incentives to uphold quality of care, including competition and patients' market freedom to secure care from whomever they choose (a bargaining power that is particularly potent where patients arrange for care in large groups); societal and professional values that focus upon the dignity of the individual and upon the commitment of the physician to serve the patient's needs; and legal expectations that care will measure up to professional standards.[94]

Further, it would be literally impossible to devise a health care system that did not carry adverse incentives of one sort or another.[95] The earlier system of retrospective fee-for-service reimbursement carried incentives to overpricing and excessive intervention.[96] Under current health care economics some incentives to overserve will remain, but mixed with many incentives to underserve.[97]

Still, the economic changes in medicine are powerful, and they threaten the physician–patient relationship in ways we have never before witnessed. In this complex situation, the financial reorganization of health care does not come already equipped with its own moral analysis. Just what it does mean for the physician and his practice is the subject of the rest of this volume.

NOTES

1. Goldman, 1984, pp. 236–37; McDowell, 1989, pp. 63–64, 71–72; Hyman and Williamson, 1988, pp. 1133, 1136, 1188; Blumstein and Sloan, 1981.

2. Eddy, 1990(a).

3. Thurow, 1984; Thurow, 1985; Eddy, 1990(a), p. 1165.

4. Roper et al., 1988; Ellwood, 1988.

5. Woolhandler et al., 1987; Relman, 1989(b), pp. 590–91; Lister, 1989; Lister, 1986; Klein, 1989; Brookes, 1989; Fisek, 1989; Iglehart, 1990.

6. Morreim, 1989(a).

7. Butler and Haislmaier, 1989, pp. 6–19, 28–31; Enthoven, 1989, pp. 37–39; Eddy, 1990(a), p. 1169.

8. Thurow, 1984; Thurow, 1985.

9. Wing, 1986.

10. Office of Technology Assessment, 1986, p. 3.

11. Iglehart, 1990; Hsiao, Braun, Ynetma et al., 1988; Hsiao, Braun, Dunn et al., 1988; Hsiao et al., 1987; Lee et al., 1989; U.S. Congress, 1989, p. H–9354 ff.

12. Egdahl and Taft, 1986, p. 60; Vladek, 1984, p. 583.

13. Mechanic, 1986; B. Brody, 1987.

14. Zuckerman et al., 1984.

15. Starr, 1982; Butler and Haislmaier, 1989, pp. 19–25.

16. Marmor, 1986; B. Brody, 1987; McDowell, 1989; Hyman and Williamson, 1988.

17. Knotterus, 1984.

18. Renlund et al., 1987.

19. Thurow, 1985, p. 611; Egdahl, 1987; Nutter, 1984, p. 918.

20. Borus, 1986, p. 1939; Mechanic, 1986, p. 38, 62–63; Feinglass, 1987, pp. 37–38; Newhouse et al., 1981; Shapiro, Ware, and Sherbourne, 1986; Meyer, 1990.

21. Patricelli, 1987, p. 77; Ginzberg, 1987, p. 1153; Butler and Haislmaier, 1989, p. 26. Some labor contracts actually established a special "hold harmless" money account for each worker, from which he could pay his higher shared costs, pocketing whatever is left at the end of the year. Employees could thus benefit from such cost containment, right alongside their employers. See Menzel, 1987, p. 71–72; Freiman, 1984, p. 86–88.

22. James, 1987(b); Butler and Haislmaier, 1989, p. 27.

23. Freiman, 1984, pp. 87–88; Mechanic, 1986, pp. 62–63; Goldsmith, 1986, pp. 3272–73; Patricelli 1987, pp. 76–77.

24. Gabel et al., 1987.

25. Wing, 1986, p. 675; Shenkin, 1986, p. 95; Butler and Haislmaier, 1989, pp. 26–27.

26. Demkovich, 1986.

27. Rundle, 1986.

28. Gabel et al., 1987, p. 47; Butler and Haislmaier, 1989, p. 26.

29. Winslow, 1989.

30. Relman, 1989(a), pp. 117–18; Himmelstein et al., 1989; Enthoven and Kronick, 1989(a); Enthoven and Kronick, 1989(b).

31. Kellermann and Ackerman, 1988; Kellermann and Hackman, 1988; Gage, 1987.

32. Starr, 1982; Fuchs, 1987, p. 1155; Ginzberg, 1987, p. 1153.

33. Hillman, Pauly, and Kerstein, 1989; Gabel et al., 1987, p. 57 ff.; Moore, 1979, p. 1359; Shenkin, 1986, p. 75 ff.; Brazil, 1986, p. 7 ff.; Butler, 1985, p. 347.

34. Mindell, 1988.

35. Gabel et al., 1987, p. 52 ff.; Shenkin, 1986, p. 92 ff.; Butler, 1985, p. 345 ff.; Rolph, Ginsburg, and Hosek, 1987, p. 33 ff.; Roble, Knowlton, and Rosenberg, 1984, p. 204 ff.; Reinhardt, 1986.

36. Gabel et al., 1987, pp. 50–52; Patricelli, 1987, p. 77 ff.

37. Leaf, 1984, p. 719; Capron and Gray, 1984; Maloney and Reemtsma, 1985, p. 1713; Spivey, 1984, p. 984. Note, although we will focus mainly on the economic pressures placed on physicians, hospitals and other institutions also face fiscal pressures that can create clinically significant incentives. Hospitals' DRG reimbursement, for instance, carries incentives to deliver care as efficiently and quickly as possible. Adverse incentives also loom, such as "skimming" the least-ill and best-reimbursed patients into one's own hospital, while "dumping" the sickest and poorest into public hospitals; "skimping" on services; "creeping" identified diagnoses into higher, better-reimbursed diagnostic categories; encouraging surgical or other more lucrative therapies where medical management might otherwise be preferable; "unbundling" patients' problems into multiple brief admissions instead of a single longer (less lucrative) stay; discharging patients prematurely, etc. See Simborg, 1981, p. 1602 ff.; Wennberg, McPherson, and Caper, 1984, p. 298 ff.; Kapp, 1984, p. 248; Iezzoni and Moskowitz, 1986, p. 927 ff.; Rhodes, Krasniak, and Jones, 1986, p. 157; Mechanic, 1986, p. 146; Begley, 1987, p. 109 ff.; Vladek, 1984, p. 584 ff.; Omenn and Conrad, 1984, p. 1314 ff.; Berki, 1985, p. 71 ff.; Matsui, 1985.

38. Winkleman and Hill, 1984, p. 2437–38.

39. Meyer 1987(c).

40. American College of Physicians, 1990.

41. Perrone, 1989.

42. Lubell, 1987; Jacobson and Rosenquist, 1988.

43. Scovern, 1988, p. 788.

44. Starzl et al., 1987.

45. Institute of Medicine, 1986, p. 171.

46. Halper, 1987, p. 161; Elkowitz, 1987, p. 273; Tierney, Miller, and McDonald, 1990, p. 1503.

47. Schroeder et al., 1984.

48. Soumerai and Avorn, 1990; Tierney, Miller, and McDonald, 1990.

49. Goldsmith, 1986, p. 3372; Spivey, 1984, p. 985; Institute of Medicine, 1986, p. 156; Hull, 1984; Hiatt, 1987, pp. 43–44.

50. Bock, 1988, p. 786; Hemenway et al., 1990, p. 1061.

51. Wong and Lincoln, 1983.

52. Reuben, 1984; Hardison, 1979; Wong and Lincoln, 1983; Lundberg, 1983.

53. Knotterus, 1984, p. 464; Havighurst, 1986(b), p. 266–67.

54. Berki, 1985, p. 72; Scovern, 1988; Pinkney, 1989.

55. Gabel et al., 1987, p. 51; Havighurst, 1986(a), p. 1126–27; Hershey, 1986, p. 54; Butler, 1985, p. 363.

56. *Sarchett v. Blue Shield*, 1987. For further discussion see Hall and Ellman, 1990, at p. 13 ff.

57. Butler, 1985, p. 364; Hershey, 1986, p. 54 ff.

58. Hershey, 1986, p. 54; Butler, 1985, p. 364.

59. Hershey, 1986, p. 58; Butler, 1985, p. 364–65.

60. Spitz, 1987, p. 62; Spitz and Abramson, 1987, p. 362.

61. Brazil, 1986, p. 7–8.

62. In 1981 Congress began to allow state Medicaid programs to institute case management as a way of coordinating as well as constraining health services for the poor. See Rosenblatt, 1986, p. 919.

63. Eisenberg 1985, p. 537–38; Iglehart, 1983, p. 978; Spitz, 1987, p. 62–63; Moore, 1979, p. 1360; Egdahl, 1987. While such gatekeepers are ordinarily installed to guard against excessive intervention, they can also be used as salesmen to promote particularly lucrative sorts of care. See Pellegrino, 1986, p. 29.

64. Veatch, 1981, p. 285.

65. Pellegrino, 1986, p. 28; Institute of Medicine, 1986, p. 156.

66. Institute of Medicine, 1986, p. 156; Butler, 1985, pp. 351, 363; Pellegrino, 1986, p. 28; Egdahl and Taft, 1986, p. 60; Moore, 1979, p. 1361; Hull, 1984; Pinkney, 1989; Blum, 1991.

67. Institute of Medicine, 1986, p. 166, 174; Gray, 1983, p. 9; Miller, 1983, p. 158; Hyman and Williamson, 1988, pp. 1143–45.

68. Capron and Gray, 1984.

69. Iglehart, 1987(b), p. 1490.

70. Scheier, 1987; Iglehart, 1987(b), p. 1490; Levinson, 1987, p. 1730.

71. Institute of Medicine, 1986, p. 156; Ellwood, Jr., 1983(a), pp. 63–64; Ellwood, Jr., 1983(b), p. 62. Indeed, physicians are owning and investing in a wide variety of health care facilities, causing concern throughout the profession. See Institute of Medicine, 1986.

72. Waldholz, 10/8/84.

73. Egdahl and Taft, 1986, p. 60.

74. Bock, 1988, p. 785.

75. Hemenway et al., 1990.

76. Gabel et al., 1987, p. 58; Hillman, 1987; Hillman, 1990.

77. Hillman, 1987, p. 1745; Scheier, 1987; Hillman, Pauly, and Kerstein, 1989.

78. Hillman, 1987, p. 1745; Egdahl and Taft, 1986, p. 60; Scheier, 1987.

79. Hillman, 1987, pp. 1143, 1147.

80. Ibid., p. 1746; Institute of Medicine, 1986, p. 157; Hillman, Pauly, and Kerstein, 1989; Hillman, 1990.

81. Hillman, 1987, p. 1745; Hillman, Pauly, and Kerstein, 1989; Hillman, 1990.

82. Berenson, 1987.

83. Hillman, Pauly, and Kerstein, 1989.

84. Brazil, 1986, p. 8; Page, 1987(a).

85. Hirshorn, 1986.

86. Meyer, 1987(a).

87. Hillman, 1987, p. 1746.

88. Scovern, 1988.

89. Morreim, 1989(a); Kusserow, 1989.

90. Salmon, 1987.

91. Brailer and Nash, 1986.

92. Council on Long-range Planning and Development, 1986, p. 3388; Glenn, Lawler, and Hoerl, 1987; Goldsmith, 1986.

93. Council on Long-range Planning and Development, 1986, p. 3384; Hernried, Binder, and Hernried, 1990.

94. Furrow, 1986, p. 991; Rosenblatt, 1986, p. 936.

95. Institute of Medicine, 1986, p. 153; H. Brody, 1987, p. 8.

96. Capron, 1986, p. 710 ff.

97. Brock and Buchanan, 1987, p. 19.

4

Fiscal Scarcity:
Challenging Fidelity

While recognizing that all these economic changes will profoundly affect health care, many physicians and bioethicists insist that physicians can and should avoid compromising their patients' welfare in the name of raising revenues or even containing costs. "Physicians are required to do everything they believe may benefit each patient without regard to costs or other societal considerations"[1]; "asking physicians to be cost-conscious . . . would be asking them to abandon their central commitment to their patients."[2] While the physician might assist in creating public or institutional resource policies, and while he occasionally must ration, as where there are too many patients for too few intensive care beds, in this traditional view he must never voluntarily say "no" to his own patient simply in order to honor third parties' economic concerns.

TRADITIONAL CONCEPTS OF FIDELITY

There are good reasons for this traditional view. It arises through a pervasive belief that physicians have special obligations of fidelity because patients are vulnerable. Health is a precondition of most life goals and projects, after all, and thus is of central importance to any autonomous person. Illness and injury often represent not merely a physical impediment to doing what one wishes, but an obstacle to clear reasoning and reflection. They can be an ontological assault on the unity of body and self, a wounding of personhood.[3]

Medical assistance renders the patient still more vulnerable. He must expose himself both physically and psychologically, laying bare the intimacies that he would otherwise reveal only to loved ones.[4] And in the process of diagnosis and treatment he may risk further harm, including permanent disability or even death, in order to regain what health he can.

43

Patients often have little choice but to submit to such exposure and risk, for medicine commonly offers their best if not only hope for improvement. And once they have opted for treatment, they must usually submit quite completely, for physicians can rarely help patients without their cooperation. Yet in that submission lies still further vulnerability from medicine's tremendous complexity and sophistication. Persons of ordinary learning are often ill-prepared even to understand their health problems and healing options, much less to evaluate the quality of care they are receiving.[5]

Physicians have always had at least some opportunity to exploit this vulnerability. Under the traditional fee-for-service system the physician not only advises the patient as to what is needed, he usually delivers the service himself—and often at a substantial fee.[6] The situation prompted George Bernard Shaw to quip:

> That any sane nation, having observed that you could provide for the supply of bread by giving bakers a pecuniary interest in baking for you, should go on to give a surgeon a pecuniary interest in cutting off your leg, is enough to make one despair of political humanity.[7]

The inequality arising from patients' vulnerabilities and from physicians' vastly superior knowledge and power can at least be ameliorated, even if not eliminated.[8] In much of our moral discourse and relevant legal literature we construe this relationship as fiduciary; that is, as a relationship in which "trust and confidence are reposed by one party in the influence or dominance of another, creating in the latter a duty to act with greater diligence and care than that required by a common negligence standard of due care."[9]

In a fiduciary relationship or, as we will call it, a relationship requiring fidelity,[10] it is said that physicians must merit patients' trust in two ways. First, patients' physical and psychological vulnerability requires that physicians be professionally competent—knowledgeable, skillful, careful, thoughtful—and that they update their knowledge and skills throughout the lifetime of their professional practice.[11]

Second, physicians must be dedicated to serving their patients' interests, even above their own.[12] In an ordinary business relationship participants are each expected to pursue self-interest, constrained only by basic rules of fairness and honesty.[13] Collectively, such self-interest is thought to be guided by an invisible hand toward the betterment of society as a whole.[14] In a fidelity relationship, on the other hand, the *caveat emptor* of business gives way to special obligations of service and loyalty. Physicians are to serve patients' needs and interests, not to exploit their vulnerability for personal gain.

This requirement of professional altruism has had two forms. On one level it has meant an effacement of self-interest[15] in which the physician is obligated to refrain from exploiting the patient and, beyond this, to promote the patient's interests, potentially even to the detriment of his own. More broadly, professional altruism has also been construed to mean that the physician must place his patient's interests above *all* others', including those of business, government, and society as a whole.[16] Let others worry about economic constraints, the argument goes; if the patient cannot count on his own physician to be his dedicated advocate, he may have no one at all.[17]

Admittedly, this latter concept of professional altruism has always been limited. Physicians have long had to divide their time among too many patients; they have always had to allocate scarce hospital beds and other commodities. And yet, until recently physicians were remarkably free to promote their patients' interests singlemindedly, regardless of the costs to others. As generous retrospective, fee-for-service reimbursement encouraged them to deliver all possible benefits, physicians' own interests mostly converged with those of their patients.[18]

Note, in discussing fidelity in this way, we are not adhering to any one particular concept of the physician–patient relationship. That relationship has come under intense scrutiny and debate in recent years, and yet virtually all proposed views of this relationship feature fidelity as a central element. The range of views includes paternalism, philanthropy, contract, contractarian, covenant, and virtue-based approaches, among others.

Prior to the mid-1960s, for instance, the prevailing concept of the physician's proper relationship with his patients was paternalism. The physician's duty was to decide what he, in his superior knowledge, skill, and wisdom, believed to be in the patient's best interests.[19] A commitment to fidelity was implicit in this approach, because the physician's focus was on the patient's welfare, not his own. The same can be said of the related position that sees the physician's efforts as philanthropy.[20] Again, the physician is dedicated to the patient's interests, even though it is presumed that his assistance is fundamentally gratuitous and not obligatory.

Contractual approaches replace the physician's prerogative to determine the patient's best interests with an insistence that the patient, as an autonomous agent, is entitled to decide for himself what values and goals will guide his care. Still, fidelity remains implicit in most versions of the contract approach. In the lone possible exception, one sees the physician as no different from the shopkeeper or the used car salesman. He is obligated to keep his promises and to refrain from fraud, but otherwise he is free to pursue his own interests.

In most renditions of the contract approach, however, the physician's obligations are seen to extend far beyond this. Though the relationship brings together two free and equal agents, one still acknowledges the serious inequality engendered by the physician's far superior knowledge and the patient's medical vulnerability. The physician therefore is said to have special fiduciary obligations, such as an affirmative obligation to come forth with information, to refrain from exploiting the patient for his own gain and, indeed, actively to promote the patient's interests above all others'.[21]

A variant of this contractual approach is contractarianism wherein, instead of seeing the physician–patient relationship as constructed of numerous actual contracts specifically negotiated between individual patients and physicians, one focuses on a hypothetical contracting process that gives rise to some basic principles to guide human interaction. In the hypothetical situation, rational contractors design the basic rules and procedures for a fair and peaceable community, knowing basic facts about human society but ignorant of the particular role that they will each play in the world that they construct. While such a process could of course give rise to a variety of plans, it would in any case require a serious measure of fidelity in the physician–patient relationship. Since anyone can expect to be a patient at one time or another, rational contractors would most likely endorse special obligations for physicians to respect patients' vulnerability.[22]

Contract-based theories have been criticized on a number of counts,[23] and further alternatives have been proposed. Pellegrino and Thomasma, for instance, argue that an excessive appeal to autonomy and contract loses sight of patients' wounded personhood,[24] and that a greater emphasis on beneficence need not return us to the paternalism long since discarded.[25] As in previous models, however, fidelity is again a major element as Pellegrino and Thomasma see physicians to have powerful special duties to help and protect their patients.

Yet another approach suggests that the physician–patient relationship is a covenant based on gift-giving, reciprocity, and a willingness "to be available to the covenantal partner above and beyond the measure of self-interest."[26] Here, too, fidelity looms large. "Key ingredients in the notion of covenant are promise and fidelity to promise . . . What a doctor has to offer his patient is not simply proficiency, but fidelity."[27]

Finally, some observers have rejected in principle all these approaches' appeals to rights, rules, and principles, in favor of an emphasis on virtues. In medicine, and in our moral lives generally, we are far less interested in whether someone follows all the rules to the letter than we are in what sort of person he is and what sorts of relationships he has. In medicine we look for such virtues as sympathy, integrity, steadfastness, honesty, and loyalty. Virtue-based models can coexist with other models of the physician–patient relationship and, again, commonly incorporate fidelity—a keeping of faith that "is properly likened to any intimate relationship, like marriage or friendship, where fidelity is the foundation and condition for the existence of the relationship."[28] "A virtue-based ethic would mandate that physicians commit themselves to obligations beyond those narrowly required by law or contract."[29]

This survey of perspectives on the physician–patient relationship is hardly exhaustive. It is sufficient, however, to illuminate one basic point: fidelity is a central element in most if not all conceptions of this relationship. And now, the new economics of medicine provokes profound challenges to our powerful, traditional notions of fidelity. These challenges particularly arise from a new kind of scarcity that has especially arisen in the past few years—fiscal scarcity.

FISCAL SCARCITY

Prior to the 1980s, limits on health care arose largely through two sources: (1) inadequate access to the health care system, either through the patient's inability to pay for care or through a regional shortage of personnel and facilities and (2) shortages of specific commodities, such as intensive care beds or hemodialysis units. Arising mainly around new or exotic technologies, serious commodity scarcities were otherwise uncommon. Government funding of capital improvements, combined with generous third-party reimbursement practices, generally meant that those who had access to the health

care system at all could expect to receive quite a full range of its benefits. As we have seen, physicians and other providers had economic
incentives to ignore costs (except where the patient himself was the
payer) and provide every possible benefit, as retrospective fee-for-service reimbursement rewarded maximal levels of intervention.[30]

In the past few years, however, a third sort of scarcity has arisen:
fiscal scarcity, a general tightening of health care dollars as government and business attempt to gain control over their skyrocketing
expenditures. As we have seen, this tightening assumes a variety of
forms—prospective payment, utilization review, preferred provider
arrangements, managed care systems—but collectively it signals a
fundamental change in the nature of the allocation decisions physicians face.

In commodity scarcity some discrete item is in limited supply,
whether because of natural limits as in the case of transplant organs,
or through sheer cost, as with positron emission tomography. The list
of patients needing that resource is usually fairly clear: only those
with severe and irreversible hepatic disease are candidates for liver
transplant. As a result, the consequences of allocation decisions are
equally clear. We know not only the exact identity of those who
receive the commodity, but also reciprocally the names, or at least the
general description, of those who do not. If Mrs. Baker is admitted to
the lone available intensive care bed, then Mr. Abel, also in need, is
not. But Mrs. Jones, recovering from pneumonia on another ward, is
unaffected. Equally important, we can also be fairly sure that if one
patient is denied the resource, some other needy person will nevertheless benefit. The difficult decision brings at least that consolation.

Because the consequences of commodity allocations are thus
fairly clear, so are the moral and medical trade-offs that must go into
those decisions. To distribute transplant organs we can assemble medical criteria to tell us which patients have the highest probability of living for what length of time, with what functional capacities and
deficits.[31] And we can identify some nonmedical values that we can
then choose either to include or to ignore. Should a criminal record
disqualify one from a transplant? Should family responsibilities or
occupational contributions count? During the early days of hemodialysis, some allocation committees decided that even after excluding on
"medical" grounds applicants who were over age forty or who suf-
fered mental illness, a surfeit of remaining candidates did require just
such clearly nonmedical considerations.[32]

Fiscal scarcity is profoundly different from this. Because every medical decision has its economic cost, literally every medical decision is now subject to scrutiny for its economic as well as its medical wisdom. Suddenly, not this or that special item, but all of medicine is an allocation issue. Every lab test. Every x-ray. Perhaps most important of all, fiscal scarcity traps the physician systematically in inescapable conflict. Bluntly: physicians serve their patients by spending other people's money and handing out other people's property. This has not always been true, because until rather recently the physician had little to offer beyond his own personal knowledge, advice, and caring. But with the emergence of costly technologies and the proliferation of economic agents who own or pay for them, the physician is increasingly caught between his patients' needs and these agents' resource limits. He is expected to make the medical (i.e., spending) decisions, because he knows what the patient needs. Yet now the economic agents whose money he has been spending are asserting control over their resources. They have created fiscal scarcity through their refusal, any longer, to pay for health care without limit. We therefore must examine the ways in which this fiscal scarcity differs from our more familiar commodity scarcity.

Unlike commodity scarcities, the consequences of fiscal allocation decisions are anything but clear. Obviously, the decision to order a $2000 course of antibiotics rather than a $2 course means that $1998 will not be available for some other patient or any other use. But beyond that, consequences are amorphous. We cannot possibly name, or even describe generically, who or what will be denied what sort of support as a result of the expenditure. The diminution of funds may constrain future decisions to some degree, though it is rare for any single spending decision to be felt discernibly even at the level of a particular hospital's finances, let alone at the statewide or national level. And the collective impact of many spending decisions does not dictate which sorts of medical care or other expenditures will be constrained for whom in the future. That is entirely a product of further decision-making.

Because the consequences of fiscal allocation decisions cannot really be specified, neither can the necessary moral or medical trade-offs be precisely identified. To prescribe a cheaper but slightly less effective antibiotic may or may not affect the patient's outcome at all; and there is no assurance that the money saved will even be used for other patients rather than returned to stockholders or taxpayers. [33]

There are other crucial differences between fiscal scarcity and commodity scarcity. Where specific commodities are at stake, it makes sense to draw a traditional distinction between issues of macro-allocation versus micro-allocation. We say that society should decide such broad (macro) questions as how much money to spend on health versus defense or education, and how much health money should go for acute care versus research or illness prevention. Physicians and other local individuals should then decide such micro questions as which particular patients will be admitted to intensive care or sent for magnetic resonance imaging. It is to this distinction that proponents of the traditional view, above, have pointed in arguing that physicians should remain aloof from basic rationing questions, even if they must occasionally allocate a scarce commodity.

In fiscal scarcity this tidy distinction has far less force. The only macro question to be answered in fiscal allocation is how many total dollars will be available in a given health care program, or for a particular technology, or to a given group of patients, or within a given hospital. After that, economic allocation is simply a matter of individual spending decisions. And those, in the main, are made by physicians, who largely control medical expenditures through their patient care decisions. Indeed, if physicians choose to be unrestrained in their ordering, they might well drive up whatever macro spending ceiling has antecedently been set. Such choices may bring a dear price to physicians or their patients, depending on incentive structures or other carrots and sticks of cost containment. But the point remains that in fiscal scarcity, virtually all allocation decisions are ultimately micro. Each is an individual decision whether to order a particular intervention (spend a sum of money) for a particular patient.[34]

The difference is particularly poignant in the clinical setting. Admittedly, it might be argued that virtually all scarcity is fiscal, since most commodities are scarce because of their cost. (The few exceptions would be items such as transplant organs that are in limited supply because of donor limitations or other nonfinancial reasons.) But at the moment of clinical decision-making the commodities are fixed. One cannot suddenly manufacture more intensive care beds or magnetic resonance imagers, so the physician must simply work with what is available. Where the problem instead is cost, the physician's predicament is quite different. It is one thing to refuse an item because there is none of it available, and quite another to say that even though it is available, it will not be used because of its expense.

Fiscal scarcity, then, is a rather new phenomenon, the product of institutional payers' and providers' need to contain their costs while seeking value for their expenditures. We have already noted that these broad economic forces are translated into specific clinical constraints through a variety of devices such as direct controls and financial incentives. As we will now see, this situation places physicians in inescapable conflicts between honoring traditional obligations of fidelity and acceding to resource constraints. We will look at four major ways in which fiscal scarcity challenges fidelity: (1) the increasing standardization of medical care; (2) stratification of resources into tiers; (3) challenges to clinical autonomy; and (4) conflicts of interest. Throughout, we will see that physicians must now routinely—not merely episodically, as in the past—balance their patients' interests against competing resource claims. Fiduciary altruism can no longer require the ostensibly complete effacement of self-interest it once did, nor the presumptive priority of one's own patients' interests over all others'.

CHALLENGING FIDELITY

Standardization of Care

As third-party payers seek value for their dollars, and as institutional providers seek to conserve their dollars while providing an acceptable product, both are asking the medical profession to examine closely its routines of care, to discern more precisely which interventions are truly of value and which are not. In the process, they are requesting physicians to adhere to streamlined efficiency guidelines or practice parameters that, it is thought, describe effective and efficient ways to deliver care for common medical situations.

The concept of clinical routines, of course, is not new. Physicians have always relied on routines of care not only to conserve time and energy, but to manage myriad details and uncertainties productively.[35] However, it is also recognized that these routines are based not just on clear data and careful reasoning, but also on habit, hunch, current fashion, and the profession's folk wisdom.[36] Further, physicians' clinical routines can vary widely from one geographic region to another, and many of these variations cannot be accounted for by incidence of illness or differences in patient population. Thus, a

> resident of New Haven, Connecticut, is about twice as likely to undergo a coronary bypass operation as is a resident of Boston;

for carotid endarterectomy, the risks are the other way around. The numbers of knee and hip replacements per capita are much more common among Bostonians, while New Havenites experience substantially higher risks for hysterectomy and back surgery.[37]

In recognition of these variations and of the sometimes limited scientific basis for clinical routines, both payers and providers, including physicians themselves, are now attempting systematically to evaluate various medical interventions and to formulate criteria for appropriate use.[38] In recent years the National Institutes of Health has sponsored a variety of consensus conferences to hone medical protocols in light of the latest research and experience. These conferences are now beginning to look at the costs as well as the effectiveness of care.[39] Beyond this, numerous medical organizations are studying medical interventions and outcomes, and formulating clinical protocols to guide medical decision-making. Thus, for example, the American College of Physicians, in collaboration with Blue Cross and Blue Shield, issued diagnostic testing guidelines for such common tests as arterial blood gas analysis, blood cultures, chest x-rays, and electrocardiograms.[40] Similarly, the American Medical Association and numerous subspecialty organizations, including the American College of Cardiology, the American College of Radiology, the American Society of Anesthesiologists, the American Academy of Orthopedic Surgeons, the American College of Obstetrics and Gynecology, and the American Psychiatric Association, are developing clinical practice standards.[41]

In like manner insurance companies, HMOs, hospitals, and other institutional providers and payers are now compiling formidable computer databases that track diagnoses, interventions, costs, and outcomes, to serve as the foundation for guidelines by which to assess both the quality and cost-effectiveness of care.[42] The Federal Government, for example, is conducting studies of assorted procedures and medical conditions, such as coronary revascularization and cholecystectomy, to ascertain medical effectiveness and cost-efficiency.[43] And numerous insurance companies have formulated their own utilization review criteria for appraising the medical necessity—and thereby the reimbursability—of medical interventions.[44]

In many ways these developments are to be welcomed. Careful study of interventions and outcomes can help to ensure that cost containment is as medically benign as possible. There are undoubtedly many ways in which physicians can reduce the quantity of their interventions without hampering quality of care, indeed improving it through reduced iatrogenesis and inconvenience.[45] Moreover, third-party payers who are no longer willing to accept "[o]racular statements by senior clinicians" as sufficient justification for paying out large sums of money[46] are entitled to some assurance that their payouts are for medical care that is genuinely needed and effective. Finally, because these protocols emerge through research and collective consensus, they can be at least somewhat less intrusive on individual patient care decisions and economically sounder than ad hoc, idiosyncratic bedside trade-offs between patients' interests and economic constraints.[47] In Chapter 5 we will explore further the appropriate role of these clinical guidelines in the moral management of medicine's changing economics. For now, however, we need to point out some serious hazards. Specifically, physicians can neither formulate nor apply such guidelines without balancing and sometimes even compromising their own patients' welfare against economic interests.

Formulating Guidelines

Some of these guidelines' hazards are methodological. They may, for example, be founded on inadequate research. Like any medical research, efficiency protocols can suffer from an oversimplified view of the problem (e.g., focusing only on one or two outcomes or therapies) or from other design flaws, inadequate data gathering techniques, insufficient data, case selection bias, excessive empiricism, or the like.[48] Beyond this, economically motivated protocols may be especially prone to ignore variables that are important but difficult to quantify, or whose inclusion might disrupt the desired economic goals.[49] Studies of cancer therapies, for instance, often examine such easily measured factors as mortality or tumor shrinkage, to the exclusion of such important matters as quality of survival.[50] Researchers hoping to find the cheapest way to achieve a preselected outcome may actually be loath to incorporate qualitative considerations if doing so would cost more money. Thus, if one drug controls angina or hypertension about as well as and far more cheaply than another, its higher rate of uncomfortable side-effects may be ignored.[51] Similarly, researchers may be tempted to focus on high-volume, high-risk acute conditions, to the neglect of chronic illnesses.[52]

Efficiency protocols may also slide over important uncertainties and contingencies. Guidelines that apply well to the general adult population, for example, may ill-serve the elderly.[53] If guidelines do not change as rapidly as medical science and clinical experience, they may be quickly outdated. And if they allow no room to consider variations in the lability and severity of patients' diseases, or education and social supports, the protocols may also pass over some of the most crucial elements in a healing relationship.[54] Indeed, if they fail to account adequately for patients' values, they may not even succeed in saving much money.[55]

The hazards of this increasing standardization of medical care run deeper. Even if based on the best and most meticulous research, these clinical protocols will not permit physicians to escape trading their patients' welfare against economic concerns. Those who formulate efficiency protocols must eliminate not just utterly useless practices, but also some interventions of at least marginal value. Though physicians have occasionally been guilty of clear wastefulness—as, for instance, admitting patients to the hospital on a Friday for an elective diagnostic workup that cannot begin until Monday—rectifying such carelessness surely will not resolve the nation's entire health care challenge.[56]

But once physicians turn to interventions of marginal value, patient care will inevitably be compromised. Not all patients' care will be impaired, for many will actually be benefited through reduced iatrogenesis and inconvenience. Nevertheless, to be of marginal benefit is, by definition, to be of some benefit.[57] The benefit may be small, as with palliative treatment of self-limited illness, or it may affect only a few. Most commonly, marginal interventions reduce diagnostic or therapeutic uncertainty—the extra laboratory test to confirm clinical findings, the screening test to detect rare but serious and treatable maladies, the wide-spectrum antibiotic to cover for unidentified organisms.[58] In most cases eliminating such interventions will do no harm. Yet some patients will be deprived of a real benefit, namely, those few whose rare disease would have been detected by the now-eliminated diagnostic "zebra-hunt," or whose therapy would have been more effective with more potent agents. We may never know in advance which patients will be harmed and which helped as efficiency protocols eliminate marginal benefits. But the fact remains that some patients' welfare will have been exchanged for the health of other patients and for the wealth of third parties.

Such trade-offs require important value judgments. To call a benefit marginal, for example, is to judge that it is intrinsically small or unimportant, or is less valuable than other uses of the limited total resources. And benefits surely are identified relative to resources. The most clearly indicated computerized tomography scan in the United States might be called an "obscene waste of money" in third-world nations, where life's most basic needs cannot always be met.[59] Yet even if we agree about that particular value judgment,[60] other decisions to label care as marginal may be more controversial. While some observers wish to label as useless the life-prolonging care of dying patients,[61] for example, some of these patients themselves might treasure even a small extension of their time.[62] This is not to say that physicians should therefore refuse to curb marginal practices. In times of resource scarcity it would be irresponsible to abdicate such essential, albeit difficult, "gray zone" decisions. Rather, the point is only that one cannot even formulate guidelines that eliminate marginal benefits without potentially incurring some genuinely unfortunate results.

Implementing Guidelines

Although they require important value judgments and will inevitably compromise some patient care, efficiency protocols can at least be formulated away from the bedside. Unfortunately, physicians' cooperation with cost containment cannot be confined to just this policy level.[63] Efficiency guidelines will not save money until they are implemented, at the bedside and in the office. And here the physician cannot escape directly saying "no" to his own patients in the name of resource conservation.

Each time an efficiency protocol would suggest suboptimal care for his patient, the physician has several choices. First, he can simply follow the protocol, refraining from any attempt to secure optimal care for his patient. In that case, he will have voluntarily done less than he could for his patient, a clear bedside trade-off.

Alternatively, he could avail himself of the flexibility that is necessarily built into such guidelines. As we noted above, no "cookbook" or computer program, however detailed, could possibly dictate exactly what should be done for each patient. Medical science is too uncertain and too rapidly changing, and patients too variable, to admit of such crisp determinacy.[64] Any guideline must therefore be tempered by the clinical judgment of a physician who personally knows the patient.[65] Thus, though barium studies of the gastrointestinal tract can normally be safely completed on an outpatient basis, a frail elderly patient may well require inpatient observation.

Such flexibility means that it is almost always possible for a physician to find some way to justify an exception for his patient, any time the guideline might propose suboptimal care.[66] Unfortunately, if the physician makes such an exception for literally every deprivation of even the smallest benefit, he will thwart the protocol completely. The very point of such guidelines is, after all, to eliminate (marginal) benefits and to distribute the resulting suboptimality of care in the most fair, medically benign way possible. If costs are to be contained, physicians must generally cooperate—at the price of voluntarily doing less than they might for some of their own patients.

In this way, the clinical guidelines that we use for fiscal scarcity are markedly different from those we use to allocate scarce commodities. Because the consequences and trade-offs of commodity decisions are fairly clear, and because decisions are episodic—required only as often as there is an available commodity-item for which too many patients compete—it is at least possible in principle to establish fairly explicit, clear criteria, and to apply them quite rigorously. One can consider whether an alcoholic ought to be denied a liver transplant,[67] and one can formulate a sorting system for allocating intensive care beds[68] or transplant organs.[69] One can also argue that these criteria need to be subjected to open public debate, since they concern macroallocation issues that properly belong to society as a whole.[70]

In contrast, the decisions of fiscal allocation are not episodic, but chronic. Every decision has its price. As a result, criteria guiding fiscal allocation ideally must cover every aspect of medical care. And each time he applies them the physician may have to engage in a moral balancing act to determine whether to accede to guidelines even though they may yield somewhat suboptimal care for his patient, or instead to dodge them and insist upon the individuality of care that can be so essential not only to good medical practice, but to honoring the patient's personal values and preferences. These private decisions cannot possibly be routinely made public. Their very frequency makes publicity unfeasible, and their specificity to individual patient circumstances would render public revelation an offense to confidentiality. Though we can and surely should discuss efficiency guidelines openly, then, it is neither possible nor desirable to make public all the real, inevitably bedside rationing decisions of fiscal scarcity.

Stratification of Resources

Traditionally, physicians have been expected to deliver a roughly uniform standard of care. Legally, they need not deliver the best of care, but they must provide at least ordinary and reasonable care. Further, this standard must be delivered regardless of whether the patient can pay. While the physician can legally refuse to accept a patient for any reason, including the patient's indigence, he may not provide substandard care to any patient accepted for care.[71] Morally, as we have seen, it has similarly been customary to expect that the physician will serve his patients' best interests without regard to others' costs.

Until recently, this requirement was not difficult to satisfy. Insurance reimbursements were generous, and providers' practice of cost-shifting (raising charges to paying patients in order to cover nonpayers) ensured that whoever had access to the health care system at all, had access to quite a full range of its benefits. Now, however, this relative equality is becoming nearly impossible to achieve. As virtually all payers and providers attempt to trim their resource consumption, the economic reorganization of health care is being felt very differently at different strata of society. In the first place, various socioeconomic groups have differing levels of health funding available. The wealthy have more than the ordinary laborer, and government funds for the poor and elderly are less generous still. At the bottom, over thirty million Americans have no health insurance.[72]

Equally important, payers are now restricting their resources exclusively to their own subscribers.[73] An insurance company may contract with a preferred provider organization, for example, to ensure that the fees it pays are not elevated to cover providers' indigent patients or their other uncompensated care. As a result the health care system, never a model of perfect equality, is becoming more sharply divided into tiers. Thurow and Reinhardt each see three tiers: "tourist class" care for people on government assistance, "business class" care for employees of corporations, and "boutique medicine" for the wealthy who can afford the private health care market.[74] One might well add a fourth tier at the bottom, for indigent patients who have no coverage from anyone.

As these tightly restricted tiers emerge, the physician may now find it impossible to provide all patients with the same basic standard of care, regardless of their economic stratum. The lesser resources of the lower tiers simply cannot support the level of care that is standard in higher tiers. This problem has already emerged as public hospitals find themselves caring for ever more indigent patients ("dumped" there from private hospitals no longer willing or able to absorb this extra uncompensated burden) on ever tighter budgets.[75] As the proliferation of costly new technologies such as lithotripsy and magnetic resonance imaging renders so-called standard care ever more costly and complex, the problem will surely be exacerbated.

This stratification of scarcity poses a serious challenge to traditional fidelity. Should we now reject our traditional insistence on a single basic quality of care? In the business world one's entitlements are directly contingent upon one's resources. "You get what you pay for" is not just a warning of *caveat emptor*, but a principle of fair exchange. Even in other fiduciary relationships it is conceded that the professional's obligations depend partly on the client's resources. The accountant may permissibly devote more and closer attention to those who pay for more of his service, even though he is obligated to promote all clients' interests with competence and integrity.[76] Why, then, has it been traditional to expect the physician to ignore financial matters?

We must again refer to patients' vulnerability. Patients have an important need that cannot be met unless they submit, sometimes at substantial personal risk, to the instruments and invasions of someone who claims to know what he is doing. The patient has no choice but to trust, yet is poorly situated to determine, until it is too late, whether his trust has been justified. It is for this reason that law and morality have both insisted that each patient is entitled to hold certain expectations, including that he will receive at least some designated minimum level of care.

Stratified scarcity now forces us to ask why, and indeed whether, that basic minimum must be the same for all patients. With the tightening of both resources and the rules for their distribution, the physician may only be able to provide fully optimal care for his lower tier patients if he is willing and able to hoard extra resources within that patient's tier or to "poach" resources from tiers above.[77] Such practices raise serious questions of justice, which we will consider in Chapter 5. For now, we need only to note that the traditional link between fidelity and equality can no longer be taken for granted. Once again, fiscal scarcity challenges traditional medical morality.

Challenges to Clinical Authority

Those who would control the costs and profits of care must control spending decisions—i.e., medical decisions. Traditionally, physicians have exercised control over medical expenditures through their power over medical decisions. After all, the physician who knows and has examined the patient is best able to determine which interventions might be medically warranted. It is the physician who informs the patient of his options, makes recommendations, and has the legal authority to prescribe medications and other interventions that require a prescription. And the physician bears legal responsibility for ensuring that the patient receives standard care. He, far more than the insurer or even the hospital, stands to be held liable wherever substandard care leads to an identifiable injury. For all these reasons the physician either controls, or at least powerfully dominates, decisions regarding money and property that usually belong to other people. He decides which of his patients will utilize a hospital bed and which of them will receive laboratory tests or physical therapy while in the hospital. Although insurers will sometimes substitute their own criteria of medical necessity for the physician's,[78] the physician still determines in large measure what costs a third-party payer will be asked to pay and, in cases where there is no third-party payer, what uncompensated costs a hospital will be expected to absorb.

Because the physician so powerfully dominates the costs that institutional payers and providers incur and because, as we have seen, the cost-conscious use of resources will require at least some compromises in patient care, some observers argue that the physician should not be the one to say no to his own patients on economic grounds. Others should say no where beneficial care must be curtailed by reason of cost.

On one version, society should be the one to say no by drawing its spending priorities more clearly.[79] However, this view is problematic. Although society can and should set basic health resource policies, legislators, bureaucrats, and judges have neither the qualification nor the authorization to make individual patient care decisions.

On another version of "let others say no," clinically knowledgeable hospital administrators or other nonphysicians should adjudicate requests for care that is not permitted by specified efficiency guidelines or that exceeds some designated threshold of expenditure.[80] As the physician pleads for his patient while others allot or deny benefits, the physician maintains unsullied his unequivocal loyalty to the patient. But at a terrible price.

He is no longer practicing medicine. Although outsiders can plausibly place some limited controls, for instance over the costliest technologies such as intensive care beds, such supervision cannot invade the daily details of care. To the extent that others determine which patients will receive how many x-rays, which laboratory or radiologic studies, or how many days of hospitalization with what intensity of nursing care, those others are literally practicing medicine in the physician's stead—without a license, at that.[81] The physician escapes saying no by becoming impotent to say yes. He is no longer clinically empowered to ensure that his patients receive the interventions they most need.

Firm guidelines and appeals procedures are initially attractive, perhaps, because they are roughly feasible in the allocation of scarce commodities. As we have seen, commodity allocation decisions are episodic, the trade-offs fairly clear, the values often nonmedical, the verdicts final. But under fiscal scarcity, all of medicine is at stake. To dictate in advance the permissible economic impact of each health care decision is to dictate the medical decisions themselves—an intrusion into clinical freedom that is medically unacceptable, morally objectionable, and legally hazardous.[82]

Only if the physician retains considerable clinical authority is he in a position to offer to each patient the interventions that each most needs. But with this resource control, in turn, come allocation responsibilities. If scarcity means that not everyone will receive what he needs, then he who controls the resources will largely determine who will receive and who must do without—including, sometimes, the physician's own patients. In sum, clinical authority can only be preserved at some cost to traditional fidelity; reciprocally, fidelity can only be kept pristine by forfeiting the authority without which one cannot practice medicine.

Conflicts of Interest

Where physicians do retain clinical authority, they face another challenge to fidelity. As noted in Chapter 3, institutional providers and financiers are creating an array of financial, professional, and personal incentives to ensure that wherever the physician retains clinical control over his practice, he nevertheless has powerful personal reasons to consider the economic implications of his decisions. In addition, physicians may voluntarily incur conflicts of interest by becoming owners or investors in a variety of facilities, ranging from pharmaceutical or medical equipment companies, to freestanding radiologic, emergency, or surgery centers, to home nursing, physical therapy, or laboratory services both in and outside of their own offices.[83]

Such arrangements are not necessarily pernicious. For one thing, it is literally impossible to establish a reimbursement system devoid of adverse incentives. "All compensation systems—from fee-for-service to capitation or salary—present some undesirable incentives for providing too many services, or too few."[84] Incentive systems may be the only, or at least the most effective way to restrain burgeoning expenditures while still leaving physicians with clinical authority. Government, after all, has many important projects besides health care; a business unable to control its production costs cannot long survive; and patients themselves have other priorities for their hard-earned wages. Furthermore, up to a point at least, reducing the intensity of medical interventions may actually improve overall quality of care through reduced iatrogenesis and inconvenience.[85] Reciprocally, preserving some of the traditional incentives to do more can help to ensure that physicians do not underserve their patients. Finally, in those cases in which a physician is an owner or investor in a medical facility, his influence on quality of care and fairness of fees may be considerably greater than it would be, were he only an employee or independent contractor.[86]

Still, virtually all of the newer financial arrangements pose more serious threats to fidelity than the fee-for-service reimbursement of the past. There, the physician's temptation to deliver excessive services was limited. Until fairly recently physicians had few interventions to offer, beyond their personal care and concern. And as technologies emerged, a relative shortage of physicians meant that each had more than enough to do. A few extra procedures would not change their income substantially. Further, in the long-term relationships of a more rural medicine, the physician had to live with the consequences of his decisions, right alongside the patient.[87] Exploitive or abusive practices thus carried strong social disincentives. Finally, patients had a safeguard. A physician cannot recommend an (unnecessary) intervention without naming it, thereby enabling the patient to ask some other physician for a second opinion.

Now, incentives of all kinds pose more serious threats to physicians' fidelity than ever before, encouraging both over- and under-service to patients. Fee-for-service conflicts have become substantially exacerbated. Costly technologies mean higher profits for physicians performing procedures, and more stringent limits on the fees paid for each procedure may encourage the physician to make up the difference by performing more procedures. Vigorous competition among both institutional and individual providers to win limited health care dollars poses further temptation to acquire the latest sophisticated technologies and then advertise vigorously to create a substantial, perhaps excessive, demand for them.

More recent incentives to hold back on costly care pose a rather different situation, with potentially very insidious hazards. Where incentives reward withholding care, the unethical physician's tool is silence, not persuasion. He never names the interventions he is withholding and, unless extraordinarily well informed, the patient never realizes that anything has been denied. The patient is poorly situated even to consider a second opinion for, at best, he could only ask the second physician the generic question whether the first is performing adequately.

The physician practicing under the new economic arrangements has incentives not only to withhold or exceed appropriate care, but also to withhold information. He may be reluctant to tell Mrs. Jones that he will earn several hundred dollars more by discharging her from the hospital today instead of tomorrow, or that his year-end income will be markedly enhanced by caring for Mr. Smith's angina himself instead of consulting a cardiologist. The patient therefore may never suspect that the physician has reasons to withhold care in the first place. Reciprocally, where the physician is an investor in a facility to which he refers his patients, the incentive toward excessive, high-priced, or even poor-quality care will be unknown to the patient unless the physician explicitly explains his financial interests.[88]

In sum, the physician's temptation to mis-serve the patient is more powerful than ever before. Aside from monetary incentives, many physicians must now pay a powerful personal and professional price in order to deliver care that previously required only their signature. They must spend many hours on telephones, haggling with utilization review personnel and assorted others who (perhaps quite appropriately) insist that physicians justify their expenditures. Physicians who care for the sickest and riskiest patients or for the chronically ill may become targets of the stiffest scrutiny, perhaps imperiling professional privileges,[89] if they do not bring their spending patterns into line with those of their peers.

In the new economics of medicine, conflicts of interest are both vexatious and inescapable. They are vexatious because as long as the physician retains his clinical authority, he is often perfectly free, in a given instance, to deliver anything a patient needs. But he still must conserve resources overall, so that whatever he delivers to one patient requires commensurate cutbacks elsewhere. The trade-offs are incremental, slippery, and deeply troubling. How badly does this patient need this x-ray? Is it really essential to prescribe a potent antibiotic for this probably viral meningitis? Because he must personally pay the price for any failure to consider economic matters, the physician will often find himself weighing his own interests against his patients'.

Fiscal scarcity, together with clinical autonomy, makes conflicts of interest inescapable for physicians. So long as resources are finite and we cannot afford to provide literally every benefit for every patient, it follows that those who control the actual clinical distribution of these limited benefits will be subjected to pressures. If economic agents such as insurers or HMOs own the resources that physicians clinically control, they will impose whatever incentives they believe are necessary to prompt the physician to think about money as well as medicine. If the physician himself owns the resources as an entrepreneur, the situation is really no different. Only the name of the owner has changed.[90]

In sum, we can no longer speak of fidelity as a benign requirement that the physician refrain from vulgar exploitation of vulnerable patients in order to line his pockets with a little extra gold, or as a simplistic command always to place the patient's interests above one's own and others'. Physicians now face systematic, often substantial personal consequences for their medical decisions. While it might once have been possible to say that the patient's interests (virtually) always warranted priority, we must now reexamine the limits of physicians' obligations.

SUMMARY

The economic overhaul of medicine requires a reevaluation of our most basic ideas about what it means for a physician to be faithful to his patients' best interests. In simpler times it required exercising one's best skill and diligence, and refraining from exploitation. As technologies emerged, generous third-party reimbursement and widespread cost-shifting ensured that these technologies were available quite freely to all patients within the health care system, even if not all patients were accepted into the system. The physician could freely promote his patients' interests by commanding, indeed in some sense commandeering, other people's money and property. If the physician admitted a patient to the hospital, his order for everything from drugs to intensive care largely determined what bills would be incurred and, depending on the patient's funding, what profits or deficits the hospital might tally for this patient's stay. Though he could not literally dictate the extent to which payers would reimburse this care, he could powerfully influence those decisions through his documented assertion of medical necessity.

The explosion of both the costs and the entrepreneurial opportunities of health care has dramatically altered this picture. If the economic agents of health care dictate precisely what interventions the physician may order for whom, they are usurping clinical authority and practicing medicine in the physician's stead. But if they leave the physician with enough clinical power to promote his patients' interests, they also leave him with powerful moral dilemmas.

The more that medical routines are standardized according to computerized data and scientific research, the more difficult it may become for the physician to insist on individuality of care for those patients whose needs exceed the "cookbook." And in every case where the patient does not fit the guidelines, the physician must decide how far to press for exceptional care. Those decisions become even more difficult where stratified scarcity hands down different "cookbooks" for patients with differing economic resources. Here, the physician may only be able to secure standard care for one underfunded patient by impinging on resources intended for other patients.

Throughout, the physician's decisions will often affect his own interests as much as the interests of patients, institutional providers, and third-party payers. In this newly complicated nexus, it becomes necessary to reexamine traditional concepts of physicians' fidelity. It is no longer plausible to demand that physicians literally always place patients' interests above their own, for in some cases this will entail a self-sacrifice that is surely beyond the call of duty. And we can no longer presume absolutely that the physician will promote his patients' interests above the competing claims of other patients, or of payers, institutional providers, and society as a whole. We must therefore consider more closely just what the physician owes his patient and, equally important, what he does not owe.[91] Having completed the foregoing work in moral diagnostics we turn, then, to the central substantive task of this volume: redefining fidelity, and ultimately medical ethics itself, in light of medicine's economic revolution.

NOTES

1. Levinsky, 1984, p. 1573.

2. Veatch, 1986, p. 38; Veatch, 1981; Abrams, 1986; Swiryn, 1986; Pellegrino and Thomasma, 1981; Angell, 1985; Hiatt, 1975; Fried, 1975; Beauchamp and Childress, 1989.

3. Pellegrino and Thomasma, 1981, p. 207 ff; Brock, 1986, p. 765; Mechanic, 1986, p. 145.

4. Capron, 1986, p. 733; Miller, 1983, p. 153.

5. Brock and Buchanan, 1987, p. 29; Miller, 1983, p. 163–64.

6. Miller, 1983, p. 161.

7. Shaw, 1911, p. 7.

8. Brock, 1986, p. 765.

9. Curran and Moseley, 1975, p. 76; Feldman and Ward, 1979, p. 81 ff; Holder, 1978, p. 225; Morreim, 1989(a).

10. Technically, the term "fiduciary" is usually restricted to certain kinds of legal relationships. Because not all scholars agree that the physician–patient relationship is fiduciary in the strictest sense, I will use the term "fidelity." See Shepherd, 1981; Feldman and Ward, 1979; Morreim, 1989(a).

11. Pellegrino and Thomasma, 1981, p. 212 ff; Gray, 1983, pp. 5–6; Holder, 1978.

12. Note, not all societies agree that the physician's primary allegiance must be to the patient. In the former Soviet Union, for example, the physician owes his first fidelity to the state. "A key problem remains the 1917 Bolshevik abolition of the Hippocratic Oath as part of an effort to do away with the 'bourgeois' approach of patient-centered medicine. It wasn't until 1971 that a Soviet doctors' oath was legislated, but it obligates the physician to submit to the state's interests first and the patient's only secondarily. 'The state is overwhelmingly focused on the health of the individual as a contributor to the economic functions of the country, rather than on the individual per se', Mr. Feshbach of Georgetown has written" (D'Anastasio, 1987, citing Murray Feshbach of Georgetown University Center for Population Research).

13. Brock and Buchanan, 1987, p. 31; Rainbolt, 1987, p. 86 ff; Veatch, 1983, p. 140 ff; Boyle, 1984, p. 783.

14. Fuchs citing Adam Smith, 1986, p. 340; Brock and Buchanan, 1987, p. 31; Jonsen, 1983, p. 1532; Luft, 1983, p. 106; Goldman, 1984, pp. 236–37.

15. Pellegrino, 1986, p. 25; Gray, 1983, p. 6; Jonsen, 1983, p. 1532; Katz, 1984, p. 89; Miller, 1983, p. 153 ff; Capron, 1986, p. 734; Kapp, 1984, p. 247; Relman, 1985, p. 750; Pellegrino and Thomasma, 1988, pp. 173–74.

16. Levinsky, 1984; Relman, 1983, p. 6; Veatch, 1981; Pellegrino and Thomasma, 1981, p. 270 ff.

17. Pellegrino and Thomasma, 1988, p. 172–89.

18. Brock and Buchanan, 1987, p. 24 ff; Relman, 1983, p. 8.

19. For a useful summary of the transition from paternalist to contractual and other models of the physician–patient relationship, see H. Brody, 1989, pp. 66–69.

20. Philanthropy is particularly well-described by May, 1975, p. 31.

21. Veatch, 1981; Veatch, 1983; Veatch, 1986. Many contractual and business relationships can carry fiduciary obligations; see, e.g., Shepherd, 1981.

22. H. Brody, 1989; Rawls, 1971(a); Rawls, 1971(b).

23. For useful summaries of such criticisms, see H. Brody, 1989; Smith and Newton, 1984; May, 1975.

24. Pellegrino and Thomasma, 1981, p. 207 ff.

25. Pellegrino and Thomasma, 1981; Pellegrino and Thomasma, 1988.

26. May, 1975, p. 35; see also May, 1983, pp. 106–44.

27. May, 1975, pp. 35, 37.

28. Smith and Newton, 1984; see also Zuger and Miles, 1987; MacIntyre, 1981.

29. Zuger and Miles, 1987, p. 1928.

30. Thurow, 1984; Thurow, 1985.

31. Starzl et al., 1987.

32. Sanders and Dukeminier, Jr., 1968; Evans, 1983(b).

33. Daniels, 1986.

34. Note, the distinction between commodity scarcity and fiscal scarcity is not equivalent to the distinction between statistical lives and identified lives. In fiscal scarcity, just as in commodity scarcity, one's decisions can affect both identified and unidentified individuals. Suppose, for example, that the physician in a crowded inner-city hospital declines to arrange for his indigent patient to receive a magnetic resonance scan from the private facility across the street on account of its cost (assume the value to the patient, though real, would be marginal, and the cost to the hospital would be too high to justify, given its dire economic condition). In this case an identified individual would be most directly affected, while other "statistical" individuals would be indirectly affected as greater fiscal resources remain for their care. In other cases a decision of fiscal allocation will have a strictly "statistical" impact on patients, as for example where a private hospital decides to set a smaller limit on the number of indigent patients it will accept.

35. Wong and Lincoln, 1983.

36. Wong and Lincoln, 1983; Egdahl, 1983; Reuben, 1984; Burnum, 1987.

37. Wennberg, 1988, p. 99; see also Wennberg, Freeman, and Culp, 1987; Wennberg, McPherson, and Caper, 1984; Wennberg, 1987; Chassin et al., 1986.

38. Relman, 1988; Riesenberg and Glass, 1989; Tarlov et al., 1989; Brook, 1989; Banta and Thacker, 1990; Woolf, 1990.

39. Mullan and Jacoby, 1985; Kosecoff et al., 1987.

40. James, 1987(a).

41. Abraham, 1989; Meyer, 1989(b); Roper et al., 1988; Kinney and Wilder, 1989, pp. 424–38; Banta and Thacker, 1990; Woolf, 1990.

42. Goldsmith, 1986, p. 3372; Epstein, 1990, p. 267.

43. Roper et al., 1988; Wennberg, 1990.

44. Melnick and Lyter, 1987; Hershey, 1986.

45. Brook, 1989; Epstein, 1990.

46. Detre, 1987, p. 624.

47. Eddy, 1990(a).

48. Eddy, 1982; Perry, 1987, p. 486.

49. Epstein, 1990.

50. Tannock, 1987.

51. Veatch and Collen, 1985.

52. Astrachan and Astrachan, 1989, p. 1511.

53. Gillick, 1987, p. 140.

54. Dans, Weiner, and Otter, 1985.

55. Wennberg, 1990.

56. Schwartz, 1987.

57. Fuchs, 1984.

58. Hardison, 1979; Reuben, 1984; Baily, 1984.

59. Aaron and Schwartz, 1985.

60. Not everyone would agree; see Woolhandler et al., 1987.

61. Angell, 1985.

62. Mitchell and Virts, 1986, p. 116.

63. Brett and McCullough, 1986.

64. Gorovitz and MacIntyre, 1976.

65. Pellegrino and Thomasma, 1981, p. 156.

66. Baily, 1986, p. 170.

67. Moss and Siegler, 1991.

68. Engelhardt and Rie, 1986.

69. Starzl et al., 1987.

70. Veatch, 1986; Fleck, 1987; Winslow, 1986; Kapp, 1984, p. 248; Pellegrino and Thomasma, 1988, pp. 185–89.

71. Morreim, 1987; Morreim, 1989(c).

72. Wilensky, 1988.

73. Fuchs, 1987, p. 1154.

74. Thurow, 1985; Reinhardt, 1985, p. 58C; Reinhardt, 1987(a).

75. Kellermann and Ackerman, 1988; Kellermann and Hackman, 1988; Nutter, 1987; Gage, 1987; Friedman, 1987.

76. Rainbolt, 1987, p. 88.

77. Morreim, 1988.

78. *Sarchett v. Blue Shield of Calif.*, 1987.

79. Abrams, 1986; Fried, 1975; Hiatt, 1975; Pellegrino and Thomasma, 1988, pp. 185–89.

80. Veatch, 1986; Veatch, 1981.

81. Hall, 1988.

82. Morreim, 1989(b); *Wickline v. State of California*, 1986.

83. Institute of Medicine, 1986; Ginzberg, 1986, p. 760; Hillman et al., 1990; Morreim, 1989(a).

84. Institute of Medicine, 1986, p. 153; H. Brody, 1987, p. 8.

85. Begley, 1987, p. 107 ff; Furrow, 1986; Brock, 1986.

86. May, 1986; Morreim, 1989(a).

87. Relman, 1983, p. 8; Brock and Buchanan, 1987, p. 24 ff.

88. Morreim, 1989(a).

89. Blum, 1991.

90. Morreim, 1989(a).

91. Note, these fundamental questions about fidelity must be asked by all physicians, not only by those practicing under the U.S. market system. In every society, health resources are finite. Because patients' needs are essentially limitless, this means that not all benefits can be provided to all people. Resources must be allocated. The rules of allocation may be explicit, as with written practice parameters, or they may be implicit, as with the informal criteria that are said to govern such technologies as hemodialysis within a nationalized system such as the British National Health Service (see Aaron and Schwartz, 1984). But in any case the physician must still decide when to accede to those rules in the name of fairness to others and when to find exemptions to them on behalf of his own patient. Similarly, whether a physician is subjected to explicit financial rewards and penalties for his resource use, or is informally admonished by fellow physicians for perceived overutilization of limited resources, he still faces personal incentives. And even in nationalized health services, stratified scarcity may appear. To the extent that citizens are permitted to purchase private health insurance, their quality of care may exceed that which is standardly provided (see Klein, 1989). To the extent that a society is geographically and socially complex, similar stratification may be found in the resources allocated to minority peoples (see Brookes, 1989).

5

The Limits and Obligations of Fidelity: Resource Use

Physicians, it would seem, are trapped between the proverbial rock and hard place. On the one hand, traditional fidelity requires them to promote their patients' best interests, using whatever resources are necessary for good medical care. On the other hand, they have lost much of their accustomed control over those resources. Similarly, traditional fidelity requires the physician to place the patient's interests above his own. And yet, as we have seen, the physician now must sometimes pay a serious personal price for doing so. As the physician exercises clinical authority over resources owned by others, those economic agents influence clinical decisions by placing the physician's own interests in jeopardy.

The simplistic, absolute ideals of the past may have been inspiring, but in the cold realities of medicine's new economics they must be reexamined. If once we could focus exclusively on the requirements of fidelity, it is time now to consider the boundaries of fidelity. That is, as we inquire what the physician owes his patient, we must also consider what he does not owe. In this chapter we will examine physicians' obligations regarding material resources, both medical and monetary. We will then, in the next chapter, reassess the physician's obligations over his own resources—his professional knowledge, skills, and effort.

THE LIMITS OF FIDELITY

Physicians' Obligations, Others' Resources

In order to redefine physicians' obligations regarding others' resources, we must look more closely at the predicament in which they find themselves. We have already seen that traditional resource expectations have outlived the physician's power to meet them.[1] Even if in a technical sense the physician can still order whatever interventions he wishes, the order quickly becomes meaningless if no one will pay to fill it.

While physicians have less direct control over resources, however, they still retain considerable indirect control. When economic agents' resource rules appear to impede care, the physician can usually find ways to "game the system"—that is, to bypass those rules while still appearing to honor them and thereby to secure resources that were not, technically at least, intended for this patient.

Gaming as an indirect resource control has two sources. First, all resource rules leave room for interpretation. They must be articulated with language, and language is inherently vague, as it uses a limited number of verbal concepts to capture the infinite variety of human experience. Reimbursement based on diagnosis-related groups, for example, requires the physician to state the patient's diagnosis. Yet in fact, it is often possible for the physician to identify his patient's condition in a variety of ways. He might describe a neurologic episode as a "probable transient ischemic attack" or as a "possible stroke,"depending on which will yield better reimbursement. Such vagueness ushers in the well-known distinction between following the letter versus the spirit of a rule. An insurer's utilization review (UR) protocols might accept a hospitalization in which a very ill patient requires close monitoring, for example, and thereby approve for payment those cases in which the patient's vital signs are being taken at least three times daily. If the physician, knowing this, orders thrice-daily vital signs on a patient who does not need them, solely to ensure UR approval, then he is honoring the letter but not the spirit of this rule.

Second, resource rules must leave flexibility for individuality of care. Medically, patients and their illnesses are too complex and diverse to be described adequately by any cookbook or computer. Any utilization guideline must leave room for atypical cases.[2] Legally and morally, physicians remain ultimately responsible for medical decisions. And as we have seen, insurers or hospital administrators who dare to dictate the daily details of care might be accused of practicing medicine without a license[3] or, at the least, could increase their own exposure to tort liability.[4] Therefore, they will usually give in to the physician who insists that his patient needs some particular intervention[5] or else will negotiate some mutually acceptable compromise.[6]

Between the resource rules' unavoidable vagueness and their necessary flexibility, then, the creative physician can invent numerous ways to game the system. Not all manipulation of resource rules counts as gaming, of course. Where resource rules are substantially ambiguous, the physician might simply select whichever fully correct description of the patient's condition will produce the most favorable application of the resource rules. For a Medicare patient with multiple medical problems, for instance, one could list her renal failure rather than her diabetes or hypertension as her principal diagnosis, thereby maximizing the hospital's DRG reimbursement. Similarly, there is nothing "gamey" about a vigorous advocacy in which the physician argues forcefully with utilization reviewers to ensure appropriate resource rulings, or uses existing appeals channels to protest inappropriate decisions.

Gaming begins when the physician pushes harder against a proper fit between language and reality as he attempts to avoid a restriction that the rule is intended to impose, or to secure a reimbursement that the rule intends not to provide. To bypass the rules in this way the physician may "fudge," using florid descriptions to exaggerate the seriousness of the patient's condition to a UR officer who has been reluctant to authorize hospitalization;[7] or he might install an intravenous line in a patient who has no need for IV medication, solely to ensure such a UR authorization. There are many methods and degrees, short of outright lying, and many physicians have expressed willingness to resort to such tactics on occasion.[8]

At the extreme, the stretch and push of fudging passes into the flagrant dishonesty of fraud. The plastic surgeon may say that this patient's rhinoplasty was "necessitated" by a (fictitious) ski accident. The internist may file claims for tests that were never performed or for patients who do not exist, or he may secure payment several times for a single procedure.[9]

Gaming the System: Reasons For

Gaming is not only quite easily available. It is now sorely tempting, because it appears to offer escape from an impossible situation. Gaming enables the physician to secure indirectly what he no longer controls directly. He still manages to extract the hospital admission or the costlier therapy, despite third parties' refusals or reluctance.

Gaming is particularly tempting in two basic kinds of situation. First, and probably most fundamentally, the patient may have no legal or economic entitlement to medical care for which he has a clear need or perhaps even some sort of moral entitlement. Where economic or legal entitlements are medically or morally inadequate, the physician may think that it is actually his duty to game the system in order to secure resources that he believes the patient ought—technicalities aside—to receive.

Let us be more precise about these three sorts of entitlement. We may think of an economic entitlement to health care as the product of free exchanges made by citizens, singly or in groups. One pays a sum to an insurer or HMO, for example, which is then obligated to provide specified services or reimbursements. Many of these economic entitlements are also legal entitlements. To the extent that these voluntary agreements represent bona fide contracts, for example, they will be enforced by civil courts. Government health programs such as Medicare and Medicaid, and the administrative rules by which they are implemented, likewise have the force of law.

While there can thus be considerable overlap, one's legal entitlements in health care can differ from his economic entitlements. Although the physician–patient relationship is ordinarily established by mutual consent, for instance, in some cases it is not strictly contractual, as where a physician agrees to treat an indigent patient gratuitously.[10] Even lacking formal economic entitlements, however, the patient still can have legal entitlements in health care. Once the physician has accepted him for care, the physician owes him the same standard of ordinary and reasonable care that he owes all his other patients, including the use of appropriate technologies, regardless of whether the patient can pay.[11]

Economic and legal entitlements, in turn, are distinct from moral entitlements to health care. To have a legal and economic entitlement is to have at least a presumptive moral entitlement, because moral principles require that governments and voluntary contractors keep their promises. If someone has promised to provide the patient with health care, that promise has a special moral force independent of its legal or economic power. On the other hand, it is at least possible to suppose that there may be moral entitlements to health care even in the absence of any formal economic or legal entitlements. Many thoughtful observers have argued that all people have a moral right to receive at least a basic minimum of health care, even if their governments fail to recognize and enforce this right with suitable health care programs. Other commentators would go beyond this to claim that we owe all citizens not just some decent minimum of care, but equal access to good quality care.[12] The latter commentators will regard the "stratified scarcity" described in Chapter 4 to be a moral anathema.

This important question can not be resolved here, but we must at least acknowledge that when a physician believes that his society's health care distribution system is morally inadequate or unjust, he may question whether he is really obligated to abide by that system's resource rules.[13] Perhaps, he might argue, he actually has a duty to use his indirect (gaming) control over resources to secure whatever the patient needs, even if those resources would not, under a strict rendering of the applicable resource rules, be intended for this patient or for this purpose. An infant recovering from meningitis may be medically ready to leave the hospital on oral antibiotics, for example, but if his fourteen-year-old, illiterate mother is unlikely to carry out the necessary outpatient regimen, the physician may want to "find" some further "medical problem" that "requires" a longer inpatient stay. The purely medical orientation of most insurance rules leaves little room for such medically significant social problems, and the physician may feel that it is imperative to secure the necessary care by whatever devices he can. Similarly, many physicians are disturbed by insurers' traditional refusal to cover useful screening tests and other important preventive care. Patients and even payers may pay a dear price for such policies, through increased incidence and severity of illness and their attendant costs. Again, the physician may be inclined to use whatever "creative writing"[14] is necessary to ensure that the patient gets what he needs.

While in some cases patients' legal and economic entitlements may be medically or morally inadequate, in other cases they do not receive even those resources to which they are, in every sense, entitled. These situations provide physicians with their second major temptation for gaming. Some insurers have developed a truly awe-inspiring array of tactics by which to avoid or delay making the payments they owe.[15] In other cases an unsophisticated UR clerk may deny approval to reimburse hospitalization for a condition that clearly requires it, as where a patient has a clinically obvious even if atypical presentation of appendicitis. Or in some instances the physician may question the patient's health care policy at a fundamental level. An HMO may lure subscribers with promises that "we provide all the care you'll ever need," yet fail to disclose a wide assortment of coverage limits, incentive systems, and barriers to care.[16] Where there is good reason to suspect that the payer is "gaming the patient," the physician may be sorely tempted to dodge its rules.

Note, patients are not the only ones whose needs may be ill-served by resource rules. Hospitals, too, can suffer economically where payers refuse to pay, or where they must care for too many indigent patients. Likewise, physicians' fees are increasingly the targets of cost containment. We can argue that physicians need to take their own incomes seriously as a moral issue,[17] and that greed can never justify gaming. We can also agree that physicians ought to provide at least some uncompensated care for indigent patients, yet we must acknowledge that these obligations are not unlimited. It is not fair to expect providers alone to make up for society's failure to construct a comprehensive health care system.

In sum, physicians face an important challenge in the new economics of health care. Although they no longer have the authority to distribute resources that they once enjoyed, they still exert considerable indirect control. If they are to deliver high-quality care to their patients in the face of resource constraints and stratified scarcity, gaming the system appears to be an attractive resolution to their seemingly impossible situation.

Gaming the System: Reasons Against

The powerful reasons tempting the physician to game the system are offset by three important counter arguments. Gaming can violate principles of nonmaleficence, of veracity, and of justice.

Nonmaleficence

Nonmaleficence is the principle of avoiding harm. Gaming can harm the very patient it is intended to help, as sadly evidenced by the story of Pauline Stafford. In this case a patient anticipating surgery for lung cancer underwent computerized tomography to ensure that her disease had not yet metastasized to the brain. Although the scan was negative, the physician instructed his office staff to write "brain tumor" in the space marked "diagnosis" on the patient's insurance form. He knew that this insurer would not reimburse any claims for "rule out" or "screen." When the patient later received in the mail a routine statement of her insurance benefits she read the entry under "diagnosis" and concluded the worst. After two days of great anguish, Pauline Stafford hanged herself. An appellate court upheld the trial jury's award of $200,000 to her husband.[18]

Even if we argue that the immediate harm to Stafford could have been avoided if the physician had explained his creative accounting system to her ahead of time, an important harm could thereby be done to her trust for him. If he is so cheerfully willing to lie for her, perhaps he is equally willing to lie to her. He could also put the patient into a very difficult situation. If the patient finds this gaming to be ethically offensive, she faces an awkward choice. Either she must resign herself to being an accomplice to a deceit she finds morally repugnant, or she must undertake the socially very difficult task of challenging her physician's honesty. If she wishes to remain in the care of this physician, it may be extraordinarily difficult for her to express her reservations about the gaming.

Patients can be harmed in other ways. If a physician exaggerates the seriousness of a patient's condition to utilization review officers on the phone, he may be obliged to enter written exaggerations in the chart, thus jeopardizing the patient's future care. Or if a psychiatrist identifies a patient's illness according to the most serious, best-reimbursed diagnosis, he may needlessly stigmatize the patient elsewhere in life.

Other patients, too, can be harmed. If a physician gains entry for his patient into a crowded coronary intensive care unit by misdescribing the patient's exclusively exertional angina as "unstable angina," some needier patient may be directly denied admission.

The physician can even hurt himself. If an adverse medical outcome happens later to lead to litigation, even altruistically motivated "fudging" in the chart or on the insurance forms could devastate that physician's credibility before a judge or jury.

More broadly, everyone can be harmed by inappropriate gaming. Where physicians routinely game their way around an undesirable resource rule instead of openly challenging it, they help to perpetuate unwise policies instead of changing them. If insurers' refusal to cover reasonable screening tests is as medically and economically counterproductive as many physicians believe, then surely it is better to challenge this policy than to preserve it by pretending to honor it even as one skirts it.

Such harms are objectionable, not just because they are intrinsically undesirable, but because in many cases they are quite avoidable. The inclination to game is often based on empirical assumptions that commonly are, in fact, incorrect. The physician may assume, for example, that a current denial of funding constitutes a permanent denial.

In most cases, however, this is not actually true. Virtually all utilization review systems have mechanisms for appealing lower-level decisions and, more importantly, it is extremely rare for prospective review to result in a flat denial of funding for care that a physician seriously argues is necessary. Almost always the physician's original plan is either accepted after further discussion or else some mutually agreeable compromise is negotiated.[19]

Similarly, where funding actually is denied or unavailable, a physician may assume that further care for the patient is thereby precluded. This assumption, too, is often erroneous, for it may be possible to find or invent alternative options. If an elderly widow is medically ready for discharge from the hospital but lacks adequate support services at home, the better remedy is to arrange for those home services, not to hold her indefinitely in a costly inpatient facility. A bit of inventiveness in recruiting family and friends can often solve the problem, even in the absence of designated funds or formal programs for home care.

Even absent such alternatives, a denial of money does not entail a denial of care. When Medicare's DRG hospital payment has been exhausted, the patient is not automatically discharged. The denial of further funding means only that continued hospitalization must be funded from somewhere else, whether by seeking money from a charitable organization, by adding to the hospital's burden of uncompensated debt, or even by expecting the patient himself to pay where he is obligated and able to do so. Similarly, an insurer's refusal to cover well-baby care is not a denial of care to the baby, but of payment to the physician.

In these ways, the gaming that the physician may feel so urgently necessary is usually, as a matter of fact, quite avoidable. Gaming is often undertaken not because there is no other way to secure a needed resource, but because it is more obvious or convenient than searching for alternatives. But of course there usually are alternatives: one can appeal, invent, negotiate, find money elsewhere, or provide services at no cost. In this context the real moral question, as we will explore it in Chapter 6, concerns the extent to which the physician is obligated to expend such effort and to endure such impositions.

Veracity

Gaming can also offend fundamental moral values of veracity. Virtually every act of gaming involves some duplicity, because by definition gaming attempts to bypass resource rules while still appearing to honor them. We need not belabor the importance of honesty. It is a basic tenet of moral integrity, of respect for other persons, and of successful communication and cooperation in a community.[20] Further, no resource system can long survive widespread abuse and dishonesty, nor can physicians expect to retain their professional integrity or, equally important, their clinical autonomy, if they treat with duplicity those who own the medical and monetary resources essential to their patients' care.[21] While the wrong is blatant where the physician deceives for his own financial gain, it is also formidable when done to help the patient. It is therefore difficult to defend even the marginal duplicity of "fudging," and probably impossible ever to justify outright fraud.[22]

Justice

Finally, gaming can offend justice. We will consider two forms of justice: contractual justice and distributive justice.

Contractual Justice. Contractual justice, or "commutative justice" as Aristotle called it,[23] concerns fair exchange and honest dealing.[24] It concerns, therefore, the economic and legal entitlements we create through voluntary agreements. Particularly, we are interested in the contracts between patients and their third-party payers. Though in a technical sense the patient is expected to pay for his own health care, in the United States this responsibility is ordinarily most directly covered by private or government insurance. Such arrangements usually constitute formal contracts. The patient (or his employer) tenders a certain amount of money while the insurer agrees to compensate the patient (or the physician directly) for specified care. Or, in a quasi-contractual arrangement, the government agrees to cover particular services for eligible patients. These agreements are limited, however. Insurers commonly specify that they will pay only for care that is medically necessary, for instance, not for experimental care or routine health maintenance.

In important ways, the physician stands in the center of this contract between patient and payer. He usually controls the patient's access to care, particularly hospitalization and any interventions that require his prescription. And, informed consent notwithstanding, patients often accept physicians' medical recommendations with little question.[25] In this way the physician substantially determines what the insurer will be asked to pay. Reciprocally, he also bears the brunt of certifying to the payer what care has actually been delivered, and of challenging denials of precertification or reimbursement.

Because the physician exercises such power as an intermediary in the patient–payer contract, he may sometimes feel serious pressures to extract services and reimbursements that the payers are not contractually obligated to make. As we noted above, many people are uninsured, and many insurance policies do not cover important medical interventions, such as screening tests and preventive care. And payers are not always quick to provide all the benefits they do owe. Furthermore, patients sometimes exert their own leverage. As their copayments and deductibles have risen with the tide of cost containment, patients who want to keep both their money and their benefits are increasingly urging their physicians to find ways to get the insurance to pay for it.

Acceding to these pressures, however, could violate two important principles underlying contractual justice: respect for autonomy and promise-keeping. First, we must recognize that these contracts are expressions of personal autonomy. A free society permits individuals to forge their own agreements with others, with the least outside interference consistent with a similar freedom for other citizens. The individual, it is thought, is better able than government to determine what his own best interests are and how best to achieve them. Accordingly, such freedom will permit people to enter voluntarily into arrangements for providing and purchasing medical insurance or other health care plans.[26]

Invariably, such agreements are limited. The subscriber pays a designated sum of money for a specified array of services or coverage. If he wants a better package of benefits, he can shop elsewhere or negotiate for more. Where someone is a rationally competent adult, where he has had the option to accept or reject a particular health policy, where he has had choices among policies, and where he has had the opportunity to supplement that policy either through purchasing an ancillary policy or through purchasing noncovered care out of his own pocket, then it is usually reasonable to suppose that his choice of health plan does express his values and priorities. His decisions may not reflect his preferences perfectly if, for example, he did not have the opportunity to negotiate individual elements within the various policies from which he was able to choose.[27] Still, his choice is his own. If he prefers to spend his money on his bowling league rather than on preventive health care, that is his decision. It is not the place of his physician, or any other outside party, unilaterally to "correct" his decisions by stretching that health policy to encompass things that it was never designed to provide. Such stretching can ultimately raise the cost of that policy to the patient, either directly through higher cost-sharing, or indirectly through reduced salary and benefits from his employer.[28]

Neither, reciprocally, is the physician entitled unilaterally to override the autonomy of those who offer such policies in the marketplace. They, just like their subscribers, are entitled to determine for themselves what they will offer and accept in their transactions.

Second, gaming can violate the moral and legal requirement that people keep their promises. Contracts, after all, are a form of promise.[29] If those who enter into such agreements cannot expect that the agreement will be fulfilled, the very enterprise of contracting is jeopardized. More to the point for our purposes, widespread gaming represents a systematic assault on patient–payer contracts. Payers and patients necessarily draw limits on their mutual obligations. Payers cannot agree to provide literally limitless care, any more than patients can pay literally limitless premiums. The physician who systematically undermines such legitimate limits through gaming not only threatens the integrity of individual agreements, he also invites economic anarchy by assaulting the confidence with which people can make such agreements in the first place. Admittedly, keeping promises can sometimes lead to unfortunate outcomes. Contracts' limits can mean denials of funding or medical care. Yet these problems should be remedied not by covertly undermining legitimate contracts through gaming, but by openly challenging the unfortunate outcomes and renegotiating the rules that gave rise to them.

As we defend the institution of contracting, we must hasten to recognize that these arguments apply only where people have freely chosen among viable options. Those who receive care by charity or by government grant cannot always be said to have entered into any such agreements. While such cases do not always involve principles of contractual justice, however, they do invoke another form of justice: distributive justice.

Distributive Justice.   Undoubtedly the physician's most serious, morally credible temptation to game resource rules arises where patients lack an economic or legal entitlement to care to which, the physician believes, the patient is morally entitled. Such a physician may feel precious little guilt if a bit of rule-dodging spares his patient suffering, morbidity, or even mortality. If the overall distribution system seems seriously unjust, it may be difficult for him to offer respectful obeisance.

Unfortunately, we cannot so easily infer from such allegations of injustice to this moral permission to game. We must look far more closely at fundamental issues of distributive justice.

As David Hume observed, scarcity necessitates justice.[30] With limited resources and limited human benevolence, social harmony requires that fair rules of distribution determine who shall receive what, and who must do without. In the clinical setting, physicians' distributive justice questions arise from an interesting combination of moral and economic factors.

On the one hand, justice as fairness requires impartiality: everyone should be treated similarly regardless of who he is, unless there is some good reason to treat him differently.[31] On the other hand, physicians' traditional fidelity requires them to be partial, actively favoring their own patients' interests over others'.

Scarcity places the physician squarely in a conflict between these two values. Earlier we argued that the physician must strive to preserve his clinical authority, so that he can best promote his own patients' interests. But if limited resources are to be distributed justly, then physicians, who control or powerfully influence those resources, must also be willing to refrain from partiality toward their own patients, even to withhold useful resources from them if that is what fairness requires. The problem is, the physician cannot both favor his patients' interests and also distribute resources impartially. He is truly in a predicament, expected on the one hand to lavish upon his own patient the best of care regardless of the consequences for others,[32] yet simultaneously to treat that patient as the moral equal of all other patients.

Some commentators would answer this predicament by suggesting that physicians cannot ethically cooperate with resource rationing until society's broader health care distribution system itself is morally just. Specifically, only in a system that assures at least a minimum level of care and is "closed"—with fixed health care budgets—can the physician ensure that the resources he conserves in one case will actually benefit other patients, rather than reverting to taxpayers or stockholders.[33]

There are three problems with this view. First, it is simply unrealistic to suppose that physicians *can* wait until society's allocation system is just, before they begin to participate in serious cost containment. Achieving major social change takes time, even if everyone agrees what changes are needed—unlikely in the current climate. And until the changes are effected, the simple fact of resource inadequacy means that resource decisions must still be made, whether or not the system is yet just. Further, as a practical matter, we have already seen that third-party payers' incentive systems can give physicians little choice but to cooperate or to get out of medicine.

Second, even if the U.S. health care system is not strictly closed, neither is it entirely open. While the physician cannot ensure that resources saved in one instance will be devoted to other needier patients, he can still be sure in a negative sense that whatever he spends on one patient will not be available for other uses. This is particularly significant for indigent care, as governments limit their outlays for the poor and as individual hospitals place ceilings on the amount of uncompensated care they will subsidize. Here the excessive cost of one patient's care can indeed change the number and identity of future indigent patients who are accepted for care by a private hospital or other provider.

Finally, distributive justice problems arise even within systems that are closed. Though a closed system may guarantee that resources withheld from one patient will be devoted to other patients, there is no assurance in any case that the resources will be used for needier patients, or that the definition of "needier" prevailing within the health care system will be one with which one morally concurs. Thus, the physician within Great Britain's National Health Service must still consider whether to refer his sixty-year-old patient for dialysis, even though the norm may be to exclude patients that age; and he must still consider whether to place his patient on total parenteral nutrition, even though other physicians in his area might consider its use in this case to be excessive.[34]

It would seem, then, that physicians cannot simply refrain from involving themselves in the existing resource allocation system until it is morally just. But the question of gaming must still be addressed. One might argue, for instance, that even though the physician must participate in an imperfect system, he can at least ameliorate its flaws by gaming his way around them. We must reject this view, for two reasons.

The first concerns what economists call the "free rider" problem,[35] or what Garret Hardin has called the "tragedy of the commons."[36] Where some social goal cannot be achieved without essentially universal cooperation—as where a community cannot build a new school unless virtually all its citizens help to pay for it—it is in everyone's interest that all citizens do their share so that the goal will be reached. At the same time, however, it is in each individual's interest to make an exception for himself, to be a free rider, so that he can avoid his share of the burden while still enjoying the successful completion of the project.[37] Reciprocally, such situations carry an assurance problem: unless each individual can be reasonably sure that his fellow citizens are contributing their fair share, he worries that his own cooperation may be a useless sacrifice, since the goal will not be reached unless everyone cooperates.

In allocating health care, this problem arises powerfully. All resource systems are finite, since of course no private payer or government can afford to pay for literally every benefit for every subscriber. Resource limits in turn necessitate allocation rules to determine who receives and who doesn't. And these rules must generally be honored, or the allocation system will collapse.

At the same time, every such system carries the seeds of its own destruction. Resource rules are unavoidably ambiguous and flexible, as we have noted. In virtually any given instance, the physician can usually game to extract an exception to the rules for his patient or himself. But such exceptions, if routinely made, are problematic in three ways.

Where gaming extracts resources for one patient that could not be afforded for all the other patients who have similar needs, one implicitly assumes that this particular patient is somehow more important, more worthy, than those other people. This presumption violates the fairness provision of distributive justice—that no person's interests are intrinsically more important than others'. Second, the gaming physician is exploiting unfairly the cooperation of his fellow physicians. He overtly pretends to honor the rules, so that the others will believe that they have assurance of his participation. Yet covertly he bypasses them, thus dishonoring the others' faith in him.

Finally, routine gaming threatens to destroy the entire allocation system. If one physician can justify making regular exceptions on behalf of himself and his patients, so can they all. Scarce resources cannot be justly distributed unless some sort of distribution system is in place, even an imperfect one. Unless the system is morally so offensive that it should be immediately abolished, it is better to change it incrementally than to overthrow it entirely. Perhaps, as with virtually every other moral principle, one can conceive of extraordinary circumstances that could, in an odd instance, justify a deviation from the norm and warrant an act of gaming. Although such situations if rare enough would not destroy an allocation system, they should surely be carefully justified as exceptions, not routinized as practices.

Suppose, however, that one really does believe that the prevailing resource system is so seriously unjust that it truly does not deserve to survive, that one cannot ethically cooperate with it. We cannot resolve here the enormous questions about what is required for a just health care system—whether people have some sort of moral right to receive health care, whether there should be equal care for all, or whether perhaps some decent minimum would be sufficient. These issues are addressed thoughtfully by many other commentators.[38] In this volume we are particularly concerned not with broad societal issues, but with the specific moral issues facing physicians in the clinical setting. Therefore, our inquiry is not what system ought to prevail, but what the individual physician should do in response to that system. More precisely: when he believes that it is unjust, should he freely game his way around it? The question brings us to our second major reason why gaming offends distributive justice. It is fundamentally an unacceptable way of bringing social change.

The reasons require a brief but important foray into political philosophy. In any society, justice is found not just in the substantive content of its laws and policies, but in the procedures by which these are made and changed.[39] That is, justice is found not only in what the rules say, but in how those rules are made.

In health care, we can debate at length about whether Medicaid ought to embrace more of the poor, or whether for such an expansion it would be acceptable to institute a priority-based rationing system, as has been proposed in some localities.[40] In a society of such widely diverse values and beliefs as the United States, however, it is unlikely that we will ever reach anything like universal agreement on the optimal content of health care benefits—or of education, or defense, or virtually any matter of national import. For this reason, it is crucial to ensure that our procedures for deciding such matters are themselves just. It is important that all serious interests be heard and that all citizens have adequate opportunity to influence policy, even if in a given instance their views do not win the day. In any society, such avenues for peaceful politicking not only show respect for citizens' differing needs and interests, they provide for stability and continuity in society and provide an alternative to violent overthrow.

The opportunity to vote, or to write one's congressman or local newspaper, however, does not always produce the results one desires. The physician may protest irrational insurance rules or Medicare regulations at length, for example, with no result but frustration and wasted time for himself and his patients.[41] Here it becomes sorely tempting to defy the rules or to ignore them. If one is unwilling to live with the rules, and unable to change them through available procedures, one's next step may be to thwart them. But at this point we must invoke an important distinction between civil disobedience and revolutionary disobedience.

The notion of civil disobedience is of course familiar. One is reminded of Gandhi, Martin Luther King, Henry David Thoreau, and countless Vietnam war protestors. Whatever one may think about the particular political goals of such activists, the tactic of civil disobedience has a very important feature. Although the person disobeys a law in order to protest it,[42] his action remains entirely within the society's procedures for making and changing its laws and policies. His conduct is open for all to see, he accepts the consequences of the legal system, and most important of all, he permits the issue finally to be resolved through society's existing procedures for making and changing its rules. He may fight vigorously to avoid imprisonment or other penalties, but his fight is undertaken within the rules of the system. Though he violates some particular rule to protest its content, therefore, he upholds the integrity of the system as a whole.

Revolutionary disobedience is fundamentally different. In revolutionary disobedience one attempts not just to challenge or change the content of some policy, but to defy or to undermine the very ways in which such policies are made and changed. When a physician games the system in order to avoid, change, or undermine that system by extracting extra health benefits for his patients or himself, he is quietly engaging in a form of revolutionary disobedience. However altruistic the motives, he is not merely averting a particular consequence; he is waging an assault on the very existence of the resource rules and defying the procedures by which they are written and implemented. This is because gaming, unlike civil disobedience, is covert. One pretends to honor the rules while in fact undermining them by systematically thwarting their intended results. Obviously, no single act of gaming can literally overthrow an entire system of resource rules. Still, the fact remains that widespread gaming constitutes a systematic subversion of the resource rules. One may easily doubt that the United States Congress always produces wise policies, yet no citizen is presumptively entitled unilaterally to defeat those policies simply because he thinks them foolish. In a democratic society, collective questions of policy are settled by public debate and by vote, either directly or through representatives. As society has the right to limit and draw priorities among its expenditures, it is not the physician's place to undermine such decisions or the democratic process by which they were wrought.[43] It is society's task, not the physician's, to determine overall access to health care.[44]

In the final analysis, then, gaming the system cannot be endorsed. It is morally and medically hazardous and is usually unnecessary as a device by which to secure needed care for patients. What we need instead is to reevaluate fundamentally our assumptions about the relationship between physicians and patients, and to reformulate traditional expectations about physicians and their use of resources.

THE OBLIGATIONS OF FIDELITY

However vigorously we argue that physicians are neither obligated nor entitled to commandeer others' money and property, or to game the system covertly to achieve that same end, the fact remains that physicians must use resources in order to deliver adequate care to their patients. The wisest, most skilled practitioner usually can do little without the diagnostic and therapeutic tools that elevate modern medicine over witchcraft and folk healing. If the physician owes the patient good care, then somehow he has obligations regarding resources. But what are those obligations? In this section we will try to reformulate physicians' resource duties by exploring first some related concepts from law, then amending and amplifying on them to construct our moral analysis.

In law, the physician's resource obligations are encompassed under the standard of care, a duty of fidelity rooted in patients' vulnerability. The patient, often ill and usually unlearned, needs to be able to trust that the physician really has and will apply the expertise he needs. He needs, that is, to be able to count on receiving at least some minimum quality of care. When medicine itself was simple, the physician could only owe his own knowledge and skill. Over the years, however, medical competence has come to include not only the duty to keep abreast of new information, but to use appropriate technologies, such as x-rays or biopsies.

> If a physician, as an aid to his diagnosis, i.e. his judgment, does not avail himself of the scientific means and facilities open to him for the collection of the *best* factual data upon which to arrive at his diagnosis, the result is not an error of judgment but negligence in failing to secure an adequate factual basis upon which to support his diagnosis or judgment.[45]

While it is not clear just how far physicians' legal duties to use technologies actually reach (e.g., there is no precedent to require that the physician purchase the patient's prescription medications out of his own pocket), the physician is usually well-advised to use whatever technological resources are clearly part of the standard of care.[46]

Furthermore, in requiring the physician simply to "take the x-rays, or have them taken,"[47] and to keep patients in the hospital as long as is medically necessary regardless of insurers' reimbursement decisions,[48] courts have shown little or no interest in who owns the x-ray machine or hospital bed, or who must pay the staff who tend them. "Whether the patient be a pauper or a millionaire, whether he be treated gratuitously or for reward, the physician owes him precisely the same measure of duty, and the same degree of skill and care."[49] The physician is thus said not only to owe adequate technological care to his patients, but to owe this equally to all his patients.

As we have seen, this longstanding economic indifference is now untenable. It places the physician in the impossible predicament of being required to deliver resources that he no longer controls—and, in the case of law, of being exposed to potential liability for failing to do the impossible. While surely the physician has an obligation to deliver quality care, and while this obligation must at some point involve resources, we can no longer hold to the simplistic demands of the past. The law, it appears, suffers from the same economic naivete that infuses traditional moral notions of fidelity. In response, we are well-advised to adapt for our moral evaluation an approach that has been recommended elsewhere for law.[50] We should divide the standard of care—the minimum quality of service that the physician morally and legally owes to any patient whom he accepts for care—into two elements.

The first is the Standard of Medical Expertise (SME). It is the level of knowledge, skill, and diligence that the physician owes each patient. It is the portion of medical care that the physician fully controls, for it involves only his professional abilities and efforts. Thus, the physician owes it to his patient to learn his craft well and to keep abreast of new medical information. And he is obligated to examine the patient carefully, to think through the diagnostic and therapeutic questions thoroughly, and to be skillful when he undertakes surgery or other procedures.

Regarding the SME, we may plausibly retain the traditional moral and legal mandate that the physician owes the same standard of care in equal measure to every patient. The physician can never be entitled to be thoughtless, hasty, or careless just because a patient is poor. We can also retain the traditional legal expectation that this standard must be set mainly by the medical profession, since it is they who develop the information and procedures that the individual physician is expected to master. In Chapter 6 we will examine more closely the obligations, and the limits, of this first form of fidelity.

The other standard is the Standard of Resource Use (SRU), encompassing the physical and thereby also fiscal resources that physicians are expected to utilize for patients. As argued in the foregoing chapters, it no longer makes sense to expect that physicians owe the same level of resources to all their patients. That is, we must reject the long-held notion that there is only one, basically uniform, standard of resource-care that physicians owe every patient. Indeed, it is not the physician who owes the resources at all. He cannot owe what others own and control, because moral obligations can only be assigned to those capable of fulfilling them. Ought implies can. Rather, the resources owed to any particular patient are determined by the specific resource arrangement in force for that patient.

The SRU is thus established not just by physicians and their medical practices, but also by payers, by patients themselves, and by society at large. The resources owed to any particular patient, therefore, can vary from one patient to the next. To the extent that a patient has contracted with a third-party payer for financial support of his health care, the SRU owed to him is mainly a product of this agreement. He is entitled to receive what he has paid for and, if someone else has paid for better coverage, then that person is entitled to receive better.

This is not to say that the SRU should be defined only in terms of technical legal and economic entitlements. Morally we might also argue that society has an obligation to ensure that all citizens have access to at least some minimum level of health care resources. If so, then we would further argue that, although the SRU may vary, there is at least some "floor" of resources that is morally owed to every person. We need not resolve that difficult question here, for if we embrace the very idea of a divided standard of care,[51] the important move for our purposes has been made. We have acknowledged that the physician's obligations over material resources are established collectively by a number of parties, not exclusively by the medical profession's judgments about what care is optimal. In this context, then, we can begin to reformulate the physician's resource obligations. The physician is obligated not to deliver resources *per se*, but to work conscientiously within a resource nexus.

Accordingly, the physician's chief resource duty is *advocacy*, particularly economic advocacy. While we can no longer suppose that physicians are obligated to commandeer what does not belong to them, they do have powerful duties, first, to advocate vigorously on behalf of their own individual patients and, second, to advocate on all patients' behalf in order to improve resource policies.

Resource Obligations: the Patient

In medical ethics literature it is traditional to speak of advocacy as "acting in the patient's best interests."[52] It is a broad definition, often associated with an equally broad concept of traditional fidelity wherein the physician was expected to order whatever interventions would benefit the patient, regardless of costs to payers or to society. As economic rearrangements now preclude this rather simplistic view, we must reconsider what it means for a physician to be his patient's advocate.

In fact, "advocate" is properly defined as "one who pleads, intercedes, or speaks for, or in behalf of, another," or as one who assists or advises another.[53] This definition is well-suited to the new economics of medicine, for it recognizes that physicians no longer exert the nearly unilateral control over resources they once enjoyed. More often, their task is to "plead the cause" of the patient, whether to an insurance company's utilization reviewers or to the intensive care unit director. We need, then, to examine the physician's new duties of advocacy. We will look first at routine responsibilities to help secure those resources to which the patient is economically or legally entitled and, second, we will consider the extent to which this advocacy should "press the system" (short of gaming) in order to maximize the patient's access to resources.

When health care reimbursement was generous and mostly automatic, the physician's duties of economic advocacy were fairly innocuous. A signature or maybe a few brief jottings usually sufficed. Economic arrangements required little explicit discussion, and the physician was seen to have clear and direct authority over resource distribution. If the patient needed something, the physician simply ordered it.

Now, however, authority over resources involves a number of parties. It is no longer possible to rely on the implicit assumption of the past that everything would somehow be paid for. Instead, the nature and scope of the patient's access to resources must now be explicitly established, and any gaps or questions about coverage must be negotiated explicitly. Many players are involved, and the physician usually must play a central role in each phase of these economic arrangings. The patient may be legally and economically entitled to designated payments from his insurer or to receive specified care from his HMO, for example, but those entitlements will only be satisfied through established rules and procedures. The insurance claim form must be filled out, perhaps including preauthorization approvals; the HMO primary physician must authorize the consult or hospitalization in writing; the director of the intensive care unit must approve this patient's admission. And these rules and procedures typically require a physician's assistance. The patient cannot claim his insurance reimbursements unless his physician attests both to the medical necessity and to the veracity of the patient's claim. Neither can he gain access to essential care itself, such as hospitalization and medications, without the physician's prescription.

Such economic advocacy, however, has created a number of new and often annoying tasks, as physicians find their time increasingly consumed by writing documentations, making phone calls, and the like. Many physicians wonder whether these economic chores are actually an obligation, or only a favor to the patient. One is his physician, after all, not his banker.

Arguably, this economic advocacy is not an optional favor, but is now a firm obligation. Money is an essential prerequisite of health care. If the patient cannot secure access to his insurance reimbursement or to medical care itself, as in the case of HMOs, unless the physician complies with required documentation, then that cooperation is just as essential to the patient's care as a careful history and physical examination.

Interestingly, even the courts are beginning to recognize such a responsibility, as seen in the case of *Chew v. Meyer*. Herbert Chew, a steel company worker who had undergone surgery, asked his surgeon, Dr. Meyer, to document for his employer that Chew's absence from work was medically necessary. Meyer reluctantly agreed to direct his secretary to complete the necessary forms but, despite several inquiries and proddings from Chew, did not in fact sign and send the forms until after Chew was actually fired from his job for failure to furnish that very documentation. In reviewing the case, the Maryland Court of Special Appeals first pointed out that the physician's promise to complete the form constituted an undertaking that, although gratuitously made, carried a duty to discharge the promise in a proper and timely manner.

The court also found another basis for liability, even more important for our purposes. In earlier times, the court argued, the plaintiff's claim

> might well have been summarily rejected, on the basis that a physician's obligation ordinarily did not extend beyond his duty to use his best efforts to treat and cure. The traditional scope of the contractual relationship between doctor and patient, however, has expanded over the years as a result of the proliferation of health and disability insurance, sick pay and other employment benefits. Today, the patient commonly, and necessarily, enlists the aid of his or her physician in preparing claims forms for health and disability benefits. Such forms ordinarily require information possessed solely by the treating physician as well as the physician's signature attesting to the bona fides of that medical information.[54]

Therefore, the court concluded, the plaintiff had on these two grounds a "plausible cause of action for breach of contract." The physician's economic assistance to the patient is no longer a matter of beneficent voluntarism, but of obligation.

Under ordinary circumstances the actual duties of economic advocacy will be fairly straightforward, because they are usually specified by the economic agents who directly control the resources. Hence, the physician must phone for prior utilization approval; he must itemize the services for which he is billing; he must sign the insurance form; he must document in writing for the HMO why he is referring this patient to a specialist.

In some cases, however, such routine compliance will not be sufficient. If the patient is indigent, the hospital administrator may urge the physician to discharge him quickly; the physician must sometimes spend hours on the phone, perhaps only to induce a recalcitrant, by-the-book utilization review clerk to authorize payment for some minor procedure; or he may be expected to write numerous letters on the patient's behalf to help protest an inappropriate denial or delay of insurance reimbursement.[55] Defending the patient's interests can cost the physician substantial amounts of (usually unpaid) time and aggravation.[56] The question arises, therefore, just how far this duty of advocacy must be carried.

That question, in turn, must be subdivided. On the one hand, we must inquire just how much time and effort the physician must personally spend in order to maximize the patient's access to useful resources. Because this particular question concerns the physician's own personal resources (his time and energy), it is reserved for the next chapter. On the other hand, we must also consider the impact that vigorous advocacy can have on other people's legitimate claims to limited resources.

Vigorous advocacy is an important tool, a crucial alternative to the moral and medical hazards of gaming. The physician might out-haggle the UR clerk or even intimidate a local hospital administrator. Or he might contest the hospital pharmacy's formulary restrictions so forcefully that the hospital relents, not because it agrees with him but simply because the dispute has become too cumbersome or costly. Pressing the system in these ways can be enormously effective when pursued with vigor and savvy. Still, the physician who successfully presses the system on his own patient's behalf is consuming resources that will thereby be unavailable for other patients or purposes. We must therefore consider how far such advocacy may be legitimate.

Tidy formulae are not available to prescribe exact answers in ethics, any more than in medicine. We can offer at most a rule of thumb, a rule that emerges from the earlier discussion of distributive justice. As noted there, any system of resource rules requires general adherence. While it might survive the gaming of a lone violator, it will collapse if the gaming becomes widespread. Therefore, as a rule of thumb: each time the physician contemplates pressing for extra resources, he should consider what would happen if all other physicians did the same under similar circumstances. In some cases the physician must conclude that the proposed "press" is clearly unacceptable. If, for example, an indigent patient at a financially desperate public hospital demands that the physician order a computerized tomography (CT) scan of his head solely for reassurance that his ordinary tension headaches do not reflect a brain tumor, the physician should generally refuse. If there is no clinical reason to suspect a tumor, to order the CT scan anyway would clearly abuse limited resources, given the fact that at this hospital other patients who urgently need this technology must often wait for it too long already. If other physicians used such an important resource for similarly frivolous reasons, the consequences for patient care overall could be disastrous.

Reciprocally, there are cases in which a patient's need is clear and urgent. If a patient presents in the emergency room with what is almost certainly an acute abdomen requiring immediate hospitalization and surgery, yet is denied payment authorization by a utilization review clerk applying standardized computer criteria over the phone, the physician surely is warranted to haggle and harangue and, if necessary, simply to admit and treat the patient and worry about the money later. If other physicians did the same under similar circumstances, patient care would be well-served and the resource system still would not be unduly pressured. The flexibility of resource rules was made for just such situations.

Considerably more difficult are intermediate situations: the physician knows that the elderly patient recovering from pneumonia is medically ready for discharge on oral antibiotics, but unable to care for herself alone at home and unable to afford the home nursing care she will need. It becomes sorely tempting to press for a prolonged hospital stay, yet such social problems are so widespread that, if all other physicians similarly used hospitalization as their primary answer to them, the cost to the health care system and thereby to other health care priorities could be enormous. Here, it becomes urgent to search for ways to secure the goal without intruding unduly on limited common resources—whether by arranging for periodic public health nurse visits, recruiting available family and friends, arranging for meals-on-wheels, or some other remedy.

Indeed, one of the most important features of medicine's economic revolution is that it forces us to look for such alternatives, to invent new ways to deliver effective care, and to consider more carefully just which medical routines are really of value. An advocacy that answers all resource needs by pressing on the existing system is, at best, short-sighted. It is a temporizing move that resolves an individual patient's problem at the cost of failing to develop more satisfactory long-term resolutions, such as requiring patients to consider more carefully which health care they really value; creating new, less costly, more convenient ways to deliver health care; and examining more closely the institutions and rules by which care is provided and financed. This brings us to the physician's second duty of advocacy.

Resource Obligations: Society

Under the divided standard of care, the standard of resource use is established not by the medical profession alone, but by a number of parties, including patients and payers. We will discuss the role of patients and payers in Chapter 7. Here we discuss physicians' part, which is to provide the medical research, judgment, and testimony necessary for any resource policy to be medically and economically credible.

As with patient-oriented economic advocacy, this obligation is not simply a gratuitous favor that the physician does, but rather is a genuine duty. The physician's knowledge and the tools he has to offer his patients are, in an important sense, not entirely proprietary. Considerable societal investment in medical education and research suggests that, although the physician may be entitled in many ways to function as a private, even entrepreneurial, provider, still he bears an obligation to return to society some of its investment in him.[57] Helping to formulate rational resource policies is one form of such repayment.

Resource policies can require the physician's assistance in two ways. They can be insufficient, as where they do not provide for important needed care. We have seen that in the United States, many people have little or no access to health care. Alternatively, resource policies can be inefficient, as where substantial amounts of money may be spent on care that is of only marginal value, perhaps to the neglect of more important interventions.

Where resources are insufficient, physicians can act both locally and globally. Locally, they can take steps to ensure that the institutions with which they are affiliated make some provision for patients who are medically indigent. At this point an interesting, yet disturbing, tension emerges. In Chapter 4 we saw that, on the one hand, physicians need to retain some measure of clinical authority over resources if they are to be able to serve their patients adequately. On the other hand, Chapter 5 argues that physicians cannot owe their patients what they neither own nor control. In this sense they do not have clinical, practical, or moral authority over other people's money and property. Where patients bring adequate funding to their health care, this tension poses relatively little problem, because the patient with his payer can authorize the necessary funding. Where the patient has no source of payment, however, the problem looms large. Adequate care requires adequate clinical tools, but those tools may not be available if unreimbursed.

While the individual physician can hardly solve this enormous social problem single-handedly, he can take some affirmative action. He can ensure that the institutional providers with which he associates develop some reasonable provision for indigent care. To some extent, this is already the case. Hospitals, for example, must deliver a hospital-specific standard of care to patients whom they admit. They are not permitted to provide inadequate nursing services or to refuse necessary diagnostic and therapeutic services to nonpaying patients. And many hospitals built with assistance from Hill–Burton funding have an obligation to accept at least some indigent patients.[58]

Beyond this, physicians can negotiate with hospitals and other institutional providers, such as freestanding surgery or ambulatory centers, to ensure that at least some reasonable number of indigent patients will be accepted and that their care will be adequately funded. Physicians do, after all, have some leverage because they are the source of institutional providers' paying patients. Thus, the individual physician should not knowingly agree to place his patients in institutions that will, in turn, "tie his hands" and preclude him from delivering adequate care. With appropriate agreements, he can at least establish enough control over resources to support the level of clinical authority he needs to provide good care. While physicians can not unilaterally grant all patients access to care, then, they can at least try to assure their own patients access to sufficient resources.

Globally, the physician also has at least some duty to remedy insufficient resources through appropriate lobbying efforts. Because physicians are most intimately acquainted with the medical effects of resource inadequacies, they are best suited to suggest to policy makers the particular ways in which resources most need to be augmented. Though gaming the system is not an appropriate way in which to effect changes, surely vigorous lobbying is. Such policy-level advocacy has been endorsed by virtually all commentators, including those who believe that physicians should take no part in rationing at the bedside.[59] The duty is also somewhat indeterminate, however, for it is probably impossible to specify with any precision just how much effort is required, concerning which particular resource policies. It is, in that sense, a general obligation that a physician could satisfy in any number of ways.

Somewhat less amorphous is the second situation, wherein resource policies are inefficient. In the face of rising health care costs and diminishing access of many patients to receive care at all, physicians should justify their medical decisions not only by their personal opinions as professionals, but by the broader wisdom of collective research and reflection. This demand for increased accountability and standardization has arisen not only out of institutional providers' and financiers' need to keep their expenditures controlled and predictable, but as well in response to the perceived inefficiencies of medical care—overuse, high variation, wasted resources, and a lack of strict scientific foundation for many of the clinical routines of care.[60] As total dollars available for health care become more strained, it can become necessary even to draw priorities among beneficial interventions. Treatment of an alcoholic's esophageal varices may prolong his life a while, for example, but at a cost of one million dollars per year of life saved.[61] Similarly, we must wonder whether the costs of routine chest x-rays are worth their benefit of detecting previously unknown and treatable maladies in only 4% of cases.[62]

Physicians themselves find practice parameters increasingly useful. Sometimes also called clinical guidelines, they promote more economical practice, reduce cost controllers' interference in clinical decision making, and help physicians to avoid having to confront awkward economic trade-offs too many times a day. With tightened clinical routines many, though not all, of these trade-offs can be managed at the policy level.[63]

As the result of all these factors, we are now seeing a wide variety of research, conducted by consensus conferences, subspecialty organizations, and interested researchers,[64] on a wide variety of topics and technologies: carotid endarterectomy, coronary angiography and upper GI endoscopy,[65] cardiac pacemaker implants,[66] inpatient versus outpatient care of common conditions,[67] and costly new technologies such as magnetic resonance imaging (MRI) and positron emission tomography (PET) scanning,[68] to name but a few.

As noted in Chapter 4, improved practice guidelines can enhance medical care in a variety of ways. They can curb costs and enhance outcomes. And, if carefully researched, they can reduce medical uncertainty by describing more precisely the indications and outcomes of various procedures under specified conditions.

We have also identified some hazards of efficiency protocols: the dangers that they may arise from inadequate or biased research, ignore quality of life or other important considerations, or hinder the individuality of care so important in medicine.

Here we must concede that, in the end, physicians cannot avoid and generally should not resist some increased standardization of care. If costs are to be contained, physicians must participate. And as they participate, their first priority must be to reconsider their routines as a whole rather than to make ad hoc trade-offs at the bedside.[69] A collective, well-researched scrutiny of common practices is far more likely to preserve quality while conserving money. It is also less arbitrary, less intrusive into the physician–patient relationship, and easier to justify to patients and payers alike. Although in the past clinical protocols may have been "a curious mixture of thoughtful research and decerebrate routine,"[70] surely it is now time to inject as much careful and critical examination as possible into the process. In that process, it will be important to improve steadily the scientific tools for undertaking such evaluations. Improvements in statistical methods, computerized data banks, new research approaches such as longitudinal observation studies, and other evaluative techniques should enhance both the quality and the clinical utility of the resultant guidelines.[71] Beyond this, such research arguably ought also to factor in costs in a careful and explicit weighing of what care is worth its cost.[72] It will also be crucial to incorporate patients' own values and preferences. Particularly for non-life-threatening and chronic conditions, many patients prefer less invasive strategies that are less risky and also less costly than those the medical profession might otherwise routinely endorse. Unless patients' preferences are carefully incorporated, practice guidelines could result in a larger system capacity, at greater cost, than is warranted to serve patients well.[73] With good quality research it should be possible for patients, payers, and physicians together to formulate better standards of resource use.

If an efficiency-minded revision of clinical protocols is an indispensable starting point, we must also add two unfortunate clinical realities to the hazards enumerated in Chapter 4. First, even the best protocols will not exempt the physician from sometimes making difficult trade-offs between costs and care at the bedside. This point is already familiar. Second, although efficiency guidelines can reduce medical uncertainty in some ways, they may exacerbate it at other points. After all, a major reason why current practices are so inflated is physicians' uneasiness with clinical uncertainty. The extra test may confirm the clinical hunch and more definitively rule out the rare disease; the broader spectrum antibiotic is just a bit surer to eradicate the infection.[74] Similarly, the principal reason we spend so much money on the care of people in their last year of life is to pursue possibilities and to rule out rarities. We do not know for certain that these were indeed the person's final days until after the life is over.[75] As streamlined practice parameters eliminate assorted interventions as unnecessary, many physicians will feel less secure in their daily management of patients. For professionals trained to value the greatest scientific precision, this infusion of greater uncertainty will be one of the most difficult and unsettling dimensions of cost containment.

While we do not back away from our conclusion that efficiency guidelines are necessary, several suggestions can help physicians to cope with these two realities. First, these guides must be based on the best data and most careful reasoning possible.[76] They must incorporate quality of life and other important considerations, and must be continually updated and adapted to a changing medical and economic environment.[77]

Second, they must still leave flexibility for individuality of care. General guidelines are useful for managing ordinary cases, but not all cases are ordinary. Patients differ not only biologically, but in the personal values that they bring to their health care choices. A guideline that left no room for important personal differences, or that ignored clinical contingencies and uncertainties, would seriously disserve both patients and the broader society.

Third, the physician must simply learn to live with greater uncertainty. Partly this requires the simple recognition that, in medicine, risks are unavoidable.[78] And partly it means that the physician must weigh a bit differently than before two very important but diverging values in health care. Since the advent of high-technology medicine and its capacity to help patients in ways undreamed of by previous generations, physicians have tended to emphasize the value, "find and fix the problem," over medicine's earlier and more modest goal of "at least, do no harm." Otherwise stated, physicians must shift from an ethic of "use it if it might help" to "don't use it unless it quite clearly will help."[79] This new focus on diagnostic elegance and therapeutic parsimony[80] will require the physician to hone his clinical acumen more finely—to cultivate better skills in doing histories, physical examinations, and good problem-solving.[81]

Finally, the physician must help his patients to live with this somewhat greater level of uncertainty.[82] It will no longer be possible to order every remotely relevant test, just to reassure the patient or just to appear thorough or just because insurance will pay for it. Conversation, rather than technology, must become the greater tool for marginal reassurance.[83]

CONCLUSION

We began this discussion by noting that physicians are now trapped between their traditional fidelity obligations to promote the patient's best interests, including to use whatever resources are necessary, and their steadily diminishing control over those resources. We have argued that this dilemma is not to be resolved by (re)asserting control—as, for instance, by gaming—over medical and monetary resources that belong to other people. Rather, the answer lies in the other direction. We must fundamentally reformulate our traditional conception of what physicians owe their patients. They are not obligated to commandeer others' money and property just because a given patient needs it. They are not obligated to hoard, poach, cheat, lie, or game the system in order to obtain resources to which the patient is neither legally nor economically entitled. And they are not ethically authorized to undertake those tactics even where they believe that the patient is being denied a resource to which he is morally entitled. Where a physician believes that health care resources are distributed unjustly, his proper recourse is not a hasty retreat to illicit gaming that covertly undermines the resource system as a whole. Rather, he is far better advised to undertake the responsibilities that are his under the standard of resource use: he should engage in vigorous advocacy to help his patients as individuals and to improve the health care system as a whole.

It is one thing to conclude that the physician does not owe what is not his to give. More delicate is the question of how far he is obligated to give what *is* his—his personal commitment and dedication—in a system that ensures his economic conscientiousness by extracting a personal price for any deviations from the economic straight and narrow path. We turn now to this issue.

NOTES

1. Admittedly, the prescription pad and the hospital order-sheet remain fairly powerful. Hospitals and other institutional providers have obligations of their own to provide adequate care, and physicians' orders often delineate what that care should be. Similarly, insurers and other third-party payers may bear a substantial burden of justification if they wish to deny payment for services that a physician has declared to be medically necessary. For a discussion of insurers' obligations, see e.g. *Sarchett v. Blue Shield of California.* (For discussion of the legal liabilities that may be alleged where insurers fail to live up to their responsibilities, see Morreim 1990(c); Stern, 1983; Abraham, 1981.) Still, for reasons outlined in preceding chapters, this power has been substantially curtailed in recent years.

2. Morreim, 1988; Morreim, 1989(b).

3. Hall, 1988.

4. *Wickline v. State of California*, 1986.

5. Berenson, 1989.

6. Gray and Field, 1989.

7. Berenson, 1989.

8. Novack et al., 1989.

9. Rundle, 1989.

10. King, 1986, pp. 15–25.

11. Morreim, 1989(c).

12. For discussions of rights to and equality in health care, see Fleck, 1989(a); Fleck, 1989(b); Buchanan, 1984; Engelhardt, 1986; Gutmann, 1983; Dougherty, 1988.

13. Daniels, 1987; Cassel, 1985.

14. Melnick and Lyter, 1987, p. 302.

15. Grumet, 1989.

16. Hillman, 1987; Levinson, 1987; Scovern, 1988; Stern, 1983.

17. H. Brody, 1987.

18. *Stafford v. Neurological Medicine, Inc.*, 1987.

19. Gray and Field, 1989.

20. Bok, 1978.

21. Gray and Field, 1989.

22. For a discussion of one particular form of fraud—forgiveness of coinsurance—see Lachs, Sindelar, and Horwitz, 1990.

23. Benn, 1967, p. 299; Aristotle, 1985, Book V, 5.13–5.71.

24. See also Rawls, 1971(a); Rawls, 1971(b); MacNabb, 1967.

25. Miller, 1983, pp. 157, 159, 164.

26. Goldman, 1984; Engelhardt and Rie, 1988.

27. We must acknowledge that, for the most part, the individual subscriber has little opportunity to negotiate the particulars of his health care coverage with his insurer. Because such contracts are commonly offered on a "take it or leave it" basis, they are usually regarded as contracts of adhesion. However, greater levels of choice are now appearing, partly as businesses offer employees a "cafeteria" approach to benefits in which employees have an array of choices among health plans; partly as the market for supplemental insurance grows to fill the gaps left by conventional insurance plans; and partly as large groups of subscribers exercise the leverage to demand greater choice among their health plan options. We will discuss this subject further in Chapter 7.

28. See Menzel, 1990; Eddy, 1990(a), pp. 1165, 1169.

29. Fried, 1981.

30. Hume, 1888, p. 484 ff.

31. Benn, 1967, p. 299; Feinberg, 1973, p. 99; Cassell, 1981, p. 78; Rawls, 1971(b), p. 83. See also, J. S. Mills' principle of treating all persons' interests equally: 1957, p. 56; and Kant's principle of universalizability (the categorical imperative): 1785, p. 31 ff.

32. Levinsky, 1984; Hotchkiss, 1987.

33. Daniels, 1987; Cassel, 1985; Pellegrino and Thomasma 1988, pp. 185–89.

34. In Great Britain's National Health Service, cost containment is achieved nationally through a fixed health care budget, and locally through informally agreed-upon criteria for access to various health services. As a result, though no one is denied care for explicitly financial reasons, patients may have to wait rather long periods of time before receiving elective interventions such as hip replacement. Here too, however, physicians can find ways to dodge the guidelines. One can ensure that his patient is seen quickly by phoning rather than writing a consultant; by classifying the patient as urgent rather than nonurgent; by instructing the patient to go directly to the emergency room or to the consultant's office; or by simply ordering the product or service. Excessive "queue-jumping," however, could destroy the system's fragile allocation system, and tends to precipitate other physicians' corrective intervention. See Aaron and Schwartz, 1984, pp. 29 ff., 52 ff., 100 ff. For useful further criticisms of the contention that physicians should not cooperate with rationing until the distribution system is just, see Menzel, 1990, p. 7 ff.

35. Buchanan, 1985, p. 23.

36. Hardin, 1968, p. 1244.

37. Baily, 1984, p. 495.

38. See, e.g., Engelhardt, 1986; Dougherty, 1988; Menzel, 1990; Buchanan, 1984; Daniels, 1985; Daniels, 1987; Welch, 1989; B. Brody, 1987; Gutmann, 1983.

39. Engelhardt, 1986.

40. Welch, 1989; Welch and Larson, 1988.

41. Grumet, 1989.

42. Civil disobedience may be direct, as where one breaks the very law he is protesting (for example, one protests a curfew law by staying out past the curfew time); or it may be indirect, as where one obstructs traffic in order to draw attention to a government weapons program. For further discussion of this and related distinctions, see Cohen, 1989.

43. Morreim, 1985(a), p. 263–64.

44. Reinhardt, in Relman and Reinhardt, 1986, p. 213; Brock, 1986, p. 763. For example, some observers have argued that the "Robin Hood" cost shifting that has long been used to cover the care of indigent patients represents an unjust redistribution of societal wealth, a unilateral resource shifting that should preferably have been explicitly debated and resolved by society as a whole. See Graham, 1987, p. 51 ff.; Hardwig, 1987, p. 52; Miller, 1983, p. 159.

45. *Smith v. Yohe*, 1963; *Clark v. United States*, 1968; *Wilkinson v. Vesey*, 1972; *Hicks v. United States*, 1966.

46. Morreim, 1989(c).

47. *Peterson v. Hunt*, 1938.

48. *Wickline v. State of California*, 1986.

49. *Becker v. Janinski*, 1891, p. 677; Morreim, 1989(c).

50. Morreim, 1989(c).

51. For arguments on behalf of the divided standard of care, see Morreim, 1989(c).

52. Daniels, 1987, p. 71.

53. Simpson and Weiner, 1989, p. 194; Black, Nolan, and Connolly, 1983, p. 27.

54. *Chew v. Meyer* 527.2d 828 (Md. App. 1987).

55. Grumet, 1989.

56. Berenson, 1989; Grumet, 1989.

57. Pellegrino, 1987; Jecker, 1990, p. 128 (discussing the views of P. Camenisch); May, 1975.

58. Starr, 1982.

59. Levinsky, 1984; Veatch, 1986; Veatch, 1981.

60. Egdahl and Taft, 1986, p. 60; Wong and Lincoln, 1983; Wennberg, McPherson, and Caper, 1984; Wennberg, 1987; Relman, 1988, p. 1220–22.

61. Begley, 1986, p. 230 ff.

62. B. Brody, 1987, pp. 43–44.

63. Eddy, 1982, p. 343; Eddy, 1990(a); Eddy, 1990(b).

64. Mullan and Jacoby, 1985; Perry, 1987; Kosecoff, Kanouse, Rogers et al., 1987; Schwartz, 1984, p. 92 ff; Banta and Thacker, 1990; Epstein, 1990; Woolf, 1990.

65. Chassin et al., 1986; Dawson, 1987; Roper, 1988; Wennberg, 1990.

66. Greenspan et al., 1988.

67. Bowen, 1987; Siu et al., 1986, p. 1259 ff.; Goldman et al., 1988; Kemper, 1988.

68. Kent and Larson, 1988; Chalmers, 1988.

69. Morreim, 1985(b).

70. Rosenberg, 1983, p. 208.

71. Wennberg, 1988; Greenfield, 1989.

72. Eddy, 1990(a).

73. Wennberg, 1990.

74. Baily, 1984, p. 495–96; Kassirer, 1989.

75. Callahan, 1986, p. 253; Scitovsky, 1984.

76. Bowen, 1987; Patricelli, 1987, p. 79–80.

77. Tannock, 1987.

78. Mold and Stein, 1986, p. 513 ff.

79. Scheff, 1963; Mold and Stein, 1986, p. 513 ff.; Thurow, 1985, p. 613; Reuben, 1984, p. 592; Brett, 1981.

80. Pellegrino, 1986, p. 27; Pellegrino and Thomasma, 1988, p. 175.

81. Mold and Stein, 1986, p. 513 ff.; Reuben, 1984, p. 592; Moskowitz, Kuipers, and Kassirer, 1988.

82. Katz, 1984, p. 165 ff.; Suchman and Matthews, 1988; Gutheil, Bursztajn, and Brodsky, 1984.

83. Povar and Moreno, 1988, p. 421; Katz, 1984.

6

The Obligations and Limits of Fidelity: Physicians' Professional Services

In a divided standard of care the physician's central duty under the standard of resource use (SRU) is economic advocacy. No longer do we view the physician, metaphorically, as a military general commanding medicine's "troops" and "tanks." Rather, we invoke metaphors of diplomacy.[1] The physician is now the patient's "chief negotiator" in a complex concatenation of resource relationships.

Still, when we come to the other standard of care, the standard of medical expertise (SME), it might be supposed that we can nevertheless retain intact the traditional requirements that the physician devote personal attention and expertise to every patient in equal measure and that he always place the patient's interests above his own. Unlike costly technologies, the physician's own knowledge, skill, and caring are truly his to give. In a world where the physician is ever less able to deliver that which his patient needs, surely this obligation of personal, professional dedication must be more unstinting than ever.

So one might argue. In this chapter, however, we will see that even these traditional duties must be substantially modified in light of medicine's economic revolution. We must begin by recalling that economic changes have introduced new complexities into physicians' relationships with their patients. Physicians have always faced conflicts between their patients' interests and their own, of course, as for example where fee-for-service has rewarded excessive intervention. But as noted in Chapter 4, physicians' interests can now conflict with their patients' to a degree not witnessed before. While it is tempting to argue that the physician still should be unstintingly dedicated and should never place his own interests above the patient's, the matter is no longer so simple. No longer is professional altruism fulfilled merely by refraining from vulgar exploitation. Though physicians must of course remain faithful to patients' interests, at some point there must be a limit to the personal or professional sacrifices they must make in order to promote their patients' smallest benefit. Simplistic admonitions of the past will not suffice to capture the moral complexity of this new environment.

Some of the familiar values, of course, remain morally forceful. The physician still should elevate his conduct above the self-interest endemic to ordinary business relations. He must refrain from deliberately exploiting the patient to promote selfish interests. He must be willing to accept a measure of personal sacrifice in order to pursue his patients' welfare, including some risk of illness and inconvenience. Medicine is, after all, a profession to help the sick, and he who cannot tolerate the unpleasant side of this work ought not to enter the profession.[2] But beyond this, we must take a new and sober look not merely at the physician's obligations, but at the limits of those obligations. We begin by discussing positive obligations and, in the next section, their limits.

THE OBLIGATIONS OF FIDELITY

Some of physicians' affirmative obligations to patients are fairly obvious, and unchanged by economics. In accepting a patient, the physician makes certain commitments as a professional. He professes, as Pellegrino and Thomasma remind us, to offer a level of knowledge and skill that the vulnerable patient needs and rightly expects.[3] This includes, of course, the traditional duty to keep abreast of new information and technology and, more recently, to learn about the real efficacy and cost effectiveness of the interventions he proposes. Professional stagnation is incompatible with the rapidly changing technologies and economics of medicine.

The physician must also exhibit the virtues necessary to an effective healing relationship, virtues such as compassion, veracity, self-discipline, courage, and respect for the patient's dignity and autonomy.[4] He owes each patient a full measure of his thought, skill, and concern. He must not become careless, casual, or insensitive merely because the patient is poor or because the insurance coverage has expired. And he must not allow his care to be hampered by judgments about the patient's personal worth.[5]

Beyond these familiar obligations physicians have two duties that, if not actually new, now arise with new dimension and force. First, the physician owes his patient economic disclosure. The medical disclosure required for standard informed consent may be familiar, but newer duties of economic disclosure require the physician to talk about price tags and incentive arrangements, and to invite the patient to participate actively in the economic trade-offs that now pit costs against care.

Second, the physician has an obligation to minimize the conflicts of interest that can compromise his loyalty to the patient. While he cannot eliminate conflicts, the physician should take great care to ensure that his affiliations with institutional payers and providers do not unduly intrude upon his duties to his patients. We will consider each of these obligations in turn.

Economic Disclosure

Information serves three important purposes in the physician–patient relationship. First, information can be a species of property. In seeking assistance from an expert, the patient's or client's primary objective may be as much to obtain understanding—to find out what this lump is, to determine whether this contract is legally binding—as to procure specific services such as trial defense or a surgical procedure. In this sense, the information is the property of the client.[6] He has purchased it and has a right to receive it.

This purchase element further reminds us that while the physician–patient relationship is fiduciary, it is usually also contractual: the patient agrees to pay the physician a specified sum for designated services. Where the patient has not been told what he will be expected to pay, he has had no opportunity to agree, disagree, or negotiate about his side of the responsibilities in their mutual agreement. In that sense, arguably there has not yet been the meeting of minds—the offer and the acceptance—that is necessary in order to establish a contractual relationship.[7] Perhaps in the days of first-dollar coverage the physician was warranted to presume that his insured patient implicitly agreed to pay whatever charges were incurred. Now, however, such an assumption is manifestly untenable. Patients bear greatly increased economic responsibilities for their care, and providers have no right to presume that patients are willing to incur whatever unspecified debt a medical recommendation happens to carry. Rather, patients are entitled to enter knowledgeably into any such contract to purchase services from physicians or other providers.

Health care contracts usually also carry implicit expectations, for example, that the physician will try to promote the patient's interests rather than exploit his vulnerability. Where these common expectations are in jeopardy, as when the physician has a major conflict of interest or when the facilities the physician offers the patient are markedly substandard, again we would argue that physician and patient have not reached a contractual meeting of the minds unless the patient has been told of these problems.

The second function of information is to provide protection. Across fiduciary relationships in general, "inequality of knowledge . . . is precisely what triggers the fiduciary aspect of the transaction."[8] The patient's or client's relative ignorance leaves him poorly equipped not only to solve the particular problem that prompts him to seek professional help, but even to appraise the quality of service he is receiving or to decide whether he wishes to continue in the relationship. He is seriously vulnerable to poor service or to exploitation. Therefore, fiduciaries are expected affirmatively to bridge this knowledge gap.[9] As noted by the California Supreme Court in *Cobbs v. Grant*, "the patient, being unlearned in medical sciences, has an abject dependence upon and trust in his physician for the information upon which he relies during the decisional process, thus raising an obligation in the physician that transcends arms-length transactions."[10] Note, this obligation contrasts sharply with ordinary business relationships. There, the seller must of course answer the consumer's questions honestly, but he is under no particular duty to volunteer information. The consumer is presumed to know what he wants, or at least what further information he wants, and is supposed to be prepared to ask his own questions and to protect his own interests.

Third, information enhances patients' autonomy, their capacity to make their own decisions in light of their own personal goals and values. The patient who must live with both his illness and its treatment is entitled, so far as he is able, to determine for himself how best to balance the benefits and burdens of proposed medical interventions. Clearly, such decisions require information.

Until recently, this primarily meant medical information. The patient needed to know his diagnosis, his treatment options, and the medical burdens and benefits of each. Economics rarely figured into these deliberations since, as outlined in Chapter 2, third-party reimbursements were deliberately structured to insulate patients and physicians from considering costs at the time of decision-making. Now, however, physicians' disclosure obligations must expand to encompass economic as well as medical information. Although most patients do have health insurance or some other coverage, the patient is nevertheless the ultimate payer, both economically and medically.

Economically, patients pay higher deductibles, copayments, and coinsurance premiums. As medical care becomes costlier, more patients reach the upper limits of their insurance policies, after which they are responsible for all health care bills.[11] Patients also bear costs indirectly. As employees, their salaries and other fringe benefits may be compromised by the rising costs of health benefits;[12] as employers and as stockholders, they see their profits diminish for the very same reason; as consumers, they pay higher prices for goods and services when health care costs raise the costs of production; as taxpayers, they pay more for government health program benefits either through higher taxes or through reductions in other government benefits.[13]

Medically, patients pay further for the increased cost of care. A useful intervention or medication may be forgone because of its cost; a nurse may be unavailable when needed because the hospital cannot afford to hire enough staff; an HMO may deliberately institute long waits for services or long drives to inconvenient locations as deterrents to overutilization; an intensive care unit may have too few beds to accommodate the next needy patient.[14]

For these three basic reasons—information as property, protection, and autonomy—it now becomes essential to inform patients about the economic dimensions of their medical choices. The burdens of a proposed intervention are no longer solely medical, because its financial costs may cause the patient and his family hardship, or force them to forgo other, preferred plans for their money or their lives. The patient has every right to decide that another year of college for his daughter is more important than coronary artery bypass surgery for himself, or that he does not want to tap his insurance company for a costly test of marginal medical value. Even ostensibly minor expenditures are rightfully the patient's concern. He may, for instance, find a minor ailment itself easier to tolerate than the expenditure of fifty or a hundred dollars for tests or treatments.[15]

Interestingly, there is both ancient and modern agreement that physicians owe their patients some economic consideration. Hippocrates stated, "'I advise making no excessive demands, but to take into account the means and income of the patient.'"[16] More recently, the authors of a prominent medical textbook argue that

> expert physicians who care for their patients will also care about their patients' economic welfare and the financial impact of their medical care. It is not proper to abrogate responsibility for medical costs by assuming that some third-party payer will provide

coverage. It is the physician's responsibility not only to hold down costs for society overall but also to know what the costs of tests and treatments are for individual patients and how much of the cost the patient will have to bear.[17]

In particular, we need to discuss patients' need for economic information in three areas: (a) the actual costs—price tags, if you will—and payment requirements for proposed interventions; (b) the economic influences, including incentive schemes and other conflicts of interest, that may affect the physician's commitment to his patient; (c) the economic controls, limits on facilities, or other factors that may hinder the physician from offering the care he thinks desirable.

Actual Costs

Unlike nearly every other consumer transaction, health care costs are usually discussed only following performance. Whereas we deem price an essential element of any bargain, the health care consumer is provided with only one aspect of price: the provider's inquiry into whether the patient or the insurer can afford the treatment.[18]

If the patient is to be a cost-conscious health care consumer, he must know what his options will cost before, not after, he chooses which interventions he wants. He needs to know not only the costs that will come out of his own pocket, but also those that will be demanded of other payers, such as his insurer. Accordingly, physicians and other providers should disclose price information.

First, the physician must make his own expectations clear. Where he himself is to provide the particular service or product, he should tell the patient in advance what fees he intends to charge or the basis on which they will be levied, and the expected cost of ancillary services such as laboratory tests or x-rays. He will probably also need to point out that unexpected medical complications can increase these figures, and may caution that an estimate is not a guarantee. Even with such caveats, however, these discussions of fees are essential before we can agree that the patient has truly consented, informedly, to receive—to purchase—the care the physician has recommended. Obviously such conversations may be abbreviated or precluded in emergency situations, but the vast majority of medical encounters are amenable to price disclosures.

The physician should also help the patient as best he can to learn the likely costs of other interventions he prescribes. Physicians often do not know what price tag is attached, for example, to the drug prescriptions they write or the physical therapy they order, for in the past there has been little need to know. Now there is a need. It is the physician who recommends which interventions the patient should purchase, and the patient often must decide for or against the intervention during their conversation—usually without much opportunity to shop around for the best quality service at the best price. Where costs can reasonably be expected to be important to the patient, it is better to discuss them before, not after, the decision about the treatment is made. If the physician wishes to recommend a costly medication, for instance, it is better to discuss alternatives in the office, than for the patient to experience "sticker shock" at the drug store and be forced either to buy the medication at a price he does not want to pay or to forgo the drug altogether—perhaps without ever telling the physician that he did not buy it, and potentially thereby complicating future diagnostic evaluation of his persisting illness.[19] Obviously it is neither possible nor reasonable to expect the physician to know literally every price of every drug at every pharmacy in town. Yet for common medications and other typical purchases that a patient is asked to make during his health care, it is often possible for physicians to learn at least a general price range. Below we will discuss further some of the practical obstacles to economic disclosure.

Other health care providers, of course, also owe the patient economic information. Institutional providers such as hospitals, ambulatory surgery or diagnostic centers, or walk-in clinics have the same obligation as the physician to provide their respective fee structures, usual charges for common procedures, and the like. Again, medical uncertainties can create economic uncertainties. No one can predict costs for an unstable patient in intensive care or for a trauma victim in the emergency room. Still, institutional providers can and should do their utmost to provide reasonable economic information, not only prospectively, but also retrospectively to explain their sometimes impossibly complex bills.[20]

Institutional payers likewise have powerful disclosure duties. Insurers, and HMOs acting in their insurer capacity, must make clear to subscribers just what they cover and what they do not, so that patients can know what out-of-pocket responsibilities they should expect for each medical choice. Payers are beginning to satisfy this obligation somewhat better in recent years, as their prospective utilization review tells patients in advance whether the insurer will reimburse a proposed surgical procedure or hospitalization. Still, there is considerable room for improvement. Payment can be denied even after utilization reviewers have certified the care; policies can be written with confusing terms and multiple caveats; patients may have to pay costly long-distance telephone bills in order to ask specifically whether their insurance covers some particular intervention; numerous other obstacles to clear understanding and prompt payment have also been documented.[21]

Patients bear important reciprocal duties. Unless he has been accepted for gratuitous care, the patient is obligated to pay his physician or other provider, as agreed between them, for the care he receives. If he enlists outside assistance, as by purchasing third-party insurance, it is still his responsibility to pay his debts. It is therefore also his job to be aware of the requirements that his chosen insurer imposes as a condition of payment. That is, although the insurer is obligated to disclose its rules clearly, the patient is obligated to be attentive so that he can do his own part to fulfill those requirements— including, for example, to inform his physician that a proposed elective surgery will require prior utilization review. Chapter 5 proposed that the physician has duties of economic advocacy to comply reasonably with the specific tasks that the payer asks of him, such as to sign claim forms and document medical necessity. Here we add that the patient who is obligated to pay him in the first place should know how that payment will be accomplished. It would be both impractical and unreasonable to expect physicians to keep track of the many third-party payers and their virtually endless variety of payment rules.

Economic Influences

As argued in Chapter 4, physicians cannot practice medicine without conflicts of interest. Where institutional payers and providers own the medical and monetary resources of care, they will either limit the physician's clinical options (a phenomenon we will consider below) or they will leave his clinical authority intact, but influence his decisions with incentives. The physician may be penalized substantial sums of money or may lose his job if he fails to meet corporate goals for productivity and economy.[22] Or he may find his role redefined, unpleasant new tasks assigned, or unfavorable changes in his working schedule.[23]

Many emergency physicians work on a contractual basis for hospitals, health care corporations, or practice groups. Continued employment may depend in part on their ability to maximize practice revenue while minimizing uncompensated care. In California, a recognition of these pressures has prompted legislative action to protect physicians from institutional retaliation when they refuse to transfer patients in unstable condition

to public hospitals, when the institution has ascertained that this patient cannot pay for his care.[24]

Analogously, the physician–entrepreneur who owns the facility to which he refers his patients must constantly look to his motives for referring, even where he has established the facility in order to provide better care at more reasonable prices to his patients. And for virtually all physicians, such mundane matters as haggling with utilization review personnel, or contesting insurers' denials of benefits, can cumulatively cost enormous amounts of time.

One way or another, whoever furnishes medicine's costly resources is now a permanent and highly influential party in the physician–patient relationship. Patients need to know this. Since physicians can no longer protect patients by avoiding conflicts of interest, they must now protect them with disclosure.

We begin with the disclosure duties owed by people other than the physician. Where an institutional payer or provider has created an incentive system, as where an HMO withholds a portion of staff physicians' salaries in order to reward or penalize economic (im)prudence at year's end, then that institution must disclose its physician-incentives not only to current patients, but as well to prospective subscribers.

This obligation may in fact be often neglected. Advertisements to entice subscribers may give glowing assurances about breadth of coverage, ease and reliability of securing benefits, and quality of care, while downplaying or ignoring exclusions, limitations, and obstacles.[25] Interestingly, we are now seeing lawsuits in which patients allege that they have been harmed by HMOs' and other institutions' failure to disclose incentive systems.[26]

Physicians, of course, also have important duties to disclose the economic pressures that influence their decisions. First, they are obligated to disclose the conflicts of interest that they themselves have created, as where the physician–entrepreneur refers his patients to his own free-standing facility, or uses in-office laboratory equipment, or sells prescription medications from within his office. They should not only relay these economic facts to the patient, but to explain their significance and provide alternative options so that the patient can freely choose.[27]

Second, physicians must inform patients about the influences by which they have agreed to be bound. An HMO may have the initial responsibility to detail for its subscribers the incentives it places on its physicians. But the physicians in that HMO have explicitly agreed to be bound by those incentives. They have therefore chosen even if not created them, and are obligated to ensure that patients understand these economic factors that can influence their medical care.

Where an incentive operates on a global level, as year-long spending patterns yield year-end salary adjustments, a global disclosure is usually appropriate. That is, one may discharge the obligation by providing an overview of the incentives and how they function at the initiation of the physician–patient relationship, with subsequent reminders or clarifications as needed. Where incentives are decision-specific, as where the physician will receive a specific cash bonus for discharging a particular patient a day early, then so must the disclosure be equally specific. The patient is entitled to know not just that physicians are sometimes given bonuses for conserving care, but that his own physician will receive this particular sum of money for this particular decision.

Limits on Care

Sometimes the economic constraints on care are beyond the physician's control. The financially strapped inner-city public hospital may not have the lithotripter commonly available at other hospitals; its intensive care unit may deny a bed to a patient who would surely be admitted almost anywhere else; its pharmacy formulary may not carry the drug that the physician thinks would best treat his patient; or an affluent private hospital may refuse to admit an indigent patient for care, once he has been stabilized in the emergency room. Such limits are usually beyond the physician's control and yet they, too, raise disclosure issues. First we must inquire whether the physician is obligated to disclose all potentially beneficial medical options—even costly ones that exceed ordinary standards of care, and which this particular patient may be unable to afford. The second, still more difficult, issue is whether the physician must inform the patient of those instances where resource constraints actually preclude him from receiving desirable care, perhaps even confining his treatment below the prevailing standard of care. We will consider these two questions in turn.

There are several reasons to identify interventions that exceed the standard. First, to the extent that the patient is paying the physician to evaluate his condition and advise him of his options, the patient is entitled to receive all the information he has purchased. This would ordinarily encompass not only those options his insurer will reimburse, but also those he might wish to purchase on his own. Even the patient with few financial resources of his own may want at least the opportunity to try to solicit elsewhere the money that he needs for the care that he wants.

This does not mean that the physician must therefore catalog all medical options to all patients, regardless how expensive or exotic. It does little good to describe a pricey rehabilitation resort to the indigent alcoholic, or to enumerate for the destitute woman at a crowded public hospital all the wonderful amenities she would enjoy if only she could afford the private hospital across town. Rather, the physician should be guided by reasonableness—by whether there is any realistic possibility that the options in question could be arranged—and by whether the patient actually wants to know. He might thus let the patient know generally that other treatment options exist, but that they are costly and not available without special provisions to pay for them. And he can then simply ask whether the patient would like to hear more about them or wants instead simply to select among the more readily available options.

Much more difficult is the second situation, in which resource constraints preclude the physician from delivering the level of care that would be considered standard for this patient under these conditions. Thus, for example: patients with this woman's pneumonia would surely be hospitalized anywhere else, but at this crowded public hospital she will be sent away from the emergency room with outpatient antibiotics and instructions to return if her condition worsens. Or for instance: anywhere else in this town, a patient with neurological symptoms like this man's would receive an immediate computerized tomography (CT) scan, yet at this hospital the waiting time even for "stat" CT on an aging scanner is many hours. In cases like these, where a patient's care falls below recognized standards, the physician faces difficult disclosure questions.

We must address them on two levels. In one sense, it seems clear that a patient is entitled to be told about all the health care options he is entitled to receive, even if resource constraints somehow preclude his actually receiving that care. This information protects patients and enhances their autonomy by opening for them the option to pursue what is rightfully theirs. Such disclosure may also help to identify and thereby to remedy the deficits in the overall health care system.

On another level, however, we must ask precisely what care a particular patient is entitled to receive. Important discrepancies can exist between one's moral, economic, and legal entitlements, as we have seen. We might believe that everyone is morally entitled to receive at least a minimum of care, yet in fact not everyone in the United States is economically or legally entitled to receive any health care other than emergency treatment at public emergency rooms. And actual economic entitlements vary enormously under conditions of stratified scarcity. A question therefore arises. Even if we can agree that the patient is entitled to receive information about whatever care he is actually entitled to receive, on what concept of entitlement should the physician base his disclosure?

We can probably rule out basing the physician's disclosure obligation on moral entitlement. There is such deep disagreement concerning whether citizens have a moral right to health care and, if so, specifically to what care that right entitles them, that we cannot at this point say what would be the correct moral standard the physician should disclose. Furthermore, the most serious problem for disclosure does not arise in this context. The physician hardly makes an astounding revelation when he informs the uninsured patient that his access to health care is sadly limited. Rather, the greatest challenge arises where one's economic entitlements are insufficient to satisfy his legal entitlement.

Malpractice tort law in the United States continues to demand that physicians provide a standard of care that is roughly uniform for all patients and yet, as we have seen, patients' economic entitlements are now quite sharply stratified into tiers. As noted earlier, courts do not yet recognize that stratified scarcity can sometimes preclude the physician from delivering the technological level of care that is otherwise standard. Where that occurs, the physician stands to be held legally liable for failing to deliver resources that, in fact, were not really available.[28] And if under these circumstances we require the physician to disclose deficiencies in the care to which the patient is legally entitled, we may in fact be requiring him to expose himself to potential legal liability. That is, as he tells the patient that he is not delivering the prevailing standard of care, he may be inviting a lawsuit.

Unfortunately, this problem will not be resolved until malpractice law has been adjusted to recognize current economic realities. It is beyond the scope of this volume to answer this interesting and powerful jurisprudential problem, but we can at least discuss some possibilities. On one view, we should simply continue to expect physicians to deliver the same standard of care to all patients and let them bear the liability consequences, in the hope that this will inspire physicians to be more efficient and to lobby more vigorously for improved health care access for all their patients.[29] However, to expose physicians to such liability, and then to require them to disclose this to patients, would arguably be seriously unfair and counterproductive.[30]

Alternatively, we might continue to expect the physician to deliver the same basic standard of care to all his patients, but permit him to rebut that presumption where serious economic constraints beyond his control precluded him from delivering that standard.[31] While this approach is more fair than the previous one, it could be cumbersome to implement, and could still require a level of equality that may not, realistically, be possible to deliver.[32]

On another approach, we might opt for a specific legislative enactment protecting physicians where resource-based inadequacies of care are beyond their control. In fact, the state of Oregon did just this in 1989, in its law revising Medicaid services. That law is designed to expand Medicaid eligibility to encompass essentially all persons below the Federal poverty level. In order to stretch the same budget to cover this larger group of beneficiaries, however, expenditures will be made according to a list of priorities among health care services. That list, to be made and regularly updated by the Health Services Commission, will be used to guide resource allocation decisions. Where funds are inadequate, services will be eliminated in order of lowest priority.[33]

Of particular interest here, the law makes two important provisions: it requires physicians to disclose any economically necessitated inadequacies in their care; and it provides immunity for physicians in those circumstances.

Health care providers contracting to provide services under this Act shall advise a patient of any service, treatment or test that is medically necessary but not covered under the contract if an ordinarily careful practitioner in the same or similar community would do so under the same or similar circumstances.[34]

Any health care provider or plan contracting to provide services to the eligible population under this Act shall not be subject to criminal prosecution, civil liability or professional disciplinary action for failing to provide a service which the Legislative Assembly has not funded or has eliminated from its funding pursuant to section 8 of this Act.[35]

As a fourth and more global option, we could endorse a divided standard of care for law, just as we have proposed in the foregoing moral analysis. That is, we could acknowledge openly, as proposed in Chapter 5, that physicians usually neither own nor fully control the technologies and other resources that they distribute to their patients. We would thus endorse the distinction between a standard of medical expertise (SME) that physicians owe and a standard of resource use (SRU) created by contractual arrangements among patients, employers, and insurers, and by statutory arrangements among legislators and citizens. The SRU, as suggested, would be established not just by the medical profession's judgments about what care should ideally be delivered, but by patients' and payers' decisions about what level of resources is desirable and affordable.[36]

There would be several advantages to such an approach. First, it would be considerably more fair to physicians, by removing the impossible expectation that they deliver resources they do not control.

Second, the divided standard of care would acknowledge not only the existence, but also the legitimacy of at least some inequality in access to health care. True equality could only be achieved in either of two undesirable ways. To eliminate stratified scarcity by eliminating all scarcity would require literally limitless health care funding, a drain that no society could afford. Alternatively, to force all citizens to accept only that minimal level that we can afford for the poorest citizens, forbidding the more affluent to spend their own money on extra care, would unduly intrude upon personal freedom. While we might believe that the current inequalities of access are unjustifiably great, we must still conclude that at least some measure of inequality is neither morally unacceptable nor practically avoidable.[37]

Third, the divided standard is capable of acknowledging that patients themselves can and should have an important role in establishing their own standard of resource use. Much more will be said on this in the concluding chapter. For now we may simply note that, where the patient has had the opportunity to decide for himself how extensively he wants costly resources to be used for his care, the divided standard approach simply expects the physician to deliver what the patient himself has chosen.

In this context, the disclosure problem can at least be ameliorated, even if not eliminated. Where the patient has substantially set his own standard of resource use through his choice of health care plan, then the physician is a friend, not an adversary, when he discloses that available facilities do not measure up to the resources to which the patient is economically and legally entitled. In such a situation the physician is not exposing himself to liability, but rather would be acting as the patient's advocate to help him secure that to which the patient has a right. Admittedly, the matter may not always be so simple. The HMO physician who informs the patient that this HMO has poorly trained ancillary staff may open himself to repercussions from his employer. Still, the most serious legal disclosure problems can probably be avoided where patients' legal entitlements are more closely attuned to their actual economic entitlements.

Unfortunately, the fact remains that malpractice law at this time can indeed expect the physician to deliver the impossible. Indeed, one of the greatest challenges we face in this new era of medicine is to unify the now-divergent expectations placed upon physicians by law, ethics, and medicine itself. Until we achieve such coherence, however, the physician is probably best advised to keep his patient informed, but with an eye toward helping him to receive the care that he needs. A patient who is in close partnership with his physician may be less likely to seek an attorney, it is to be hoped, than the patient who discovers on his own, by a nasty surprise, that his physician "held out" on him. Indeed, in the first and most prominent lawsuit to date that concerns economically prompted denials of care, the plaintiff who believed she had been discharged from the hospital too early declined to sue her physicians, suing only the state Medicaid program that had denied funding for a longer stay.[38] The physicians, she felt, were as much victims of the system as she was.[39]

Even if we can manage the legal hazards of economic disclosure, important social hazards remain. Although they are morally necessary, these disclosures can still lead to misunderstanding and they may be socially awkward. Discussions about fees and conflicts of interest are uncomfortable for many people but, particularly in medicine where money is rarely discussed, both physician and patient may feel especially tainted by putting price tags on life and health.

A parent, for example, may be embarrassed to ask about the cost of his child's care, or ashamed to say that he cannot afford to spend the money necessary to make his child well. The patient who is told that his physician is an investor in the freestanding diagnostic center to which he is being referred may misunderstand the point of the physician's disclosure. He may suppose that the physician is depicting the center as simply an extension of his own office or he may infer that, since the physician owns it, the center must be particularly excellent. Once he realizes that the disclosure constitutes a warning, not reassurance, the patient may find it socially awkward to act on his understanding. Even if he would like to be referred to another facility, he may be reluctant to insult the physician's integrity by asking to go elsewhere; he may not want to appear to be contrary or noncompliant; he may fear that buying from the competition may hurt his physician economically or, worse yet, force him to raise his professional fees.

The physician, likewise, may feel awkward about discussing prices, incentive schemes, or inadequacies of resources. He may damage the patient's trust as he explains, "the less I do for you, the more money I take home." He may fear that a frank discussion about costs could prompt the patient to believe that the physician cares more about being paid than about curing the illness.

The problem runs deep. Fiscal scarcity ensures the persistence and the pervasiveness of devices to contain costs and boost revenues. Openly disclosing costs and conflicts of interest to patients, many of whom are quite unaccustomed to thinking about money and medicine in the same breath, may seriously undermine their faith in the medical community in general and in their own physician in particular. Yet a failure to disclose economic information leaves patients even more vulnerable than ever to exploitation or inferior care. As the ultimate payers for health care—both economically and medically—it is now time for patients to become systematically and intimately involved in weighing the medical benefits against the economic burdens of care.

There are several ways in which the awkwardness of economic discussions can be ameliorated. First, it is necessary for patients and physicians to revise their mutual expectations. Disclosures about high prices, conflicts of interest, or inadequacies of care are sure to be distressing sometimes, and yet neither physicians nor patients can prepare themselves to make intelligent decisions about health care and its resources unless they know, quite realistically, just what situation they face. Patients need to recognize that physicians can no longer deliver the unlimited resources and unstinting devotion of the past. As we will propose in Chapter 7, patients need to be far more intimately involved in choosing and shaping their health care coverage. In order to do this, they need to be informed all along about the economic dimensions of their care. In the same vein, physicians need to recognize that institutional payers' and providers' legitimate requirements and constraints must now factor explicitly into the physician's decisions and his conversations with his patients.[40]

Second, the physician needs to bring to economic matters the same careful communication skills that he must already develop for other difficult conversations about death, disease, and deviance. He may, for example, need to explain why he is broaching cost issues before he actually discusses prices: "Most patients are embarrassed to ask about money matters, but I know that you may be just as worried about how much this will cost as about how much it'll hurt. So I'll be glad to discuss that with you, if you want, or to have one of our office staff go over all the costs."

Even conflicts of interest can be revealed in fairly benign ways: "Mrs. Jones, there are several places you can get your mammogram. One is very near your home, but they're a bit more expensive than the one on the east side of town; there's another that has evening hours of operation, in case that fits your work schedule better. You should also know that I have an investment interest in one of them. I don't want you to feel obligated to go there, though, so I'll only tell you which one it is if you'd actually like to know. The important thing is that we choose the one that best fits your needs."

Third, there are some very practical tactics that can make economic disclosure—and economic advocacy, as described in Chapter 5—considerably easier. Many physicians will find it useful to hire special office staff to help carry out the duties of economic advocacy and disclosure—informing patients about billing and pricing practices, phoning insurers for utilization approval, helping to challenge reimbursement denials, and the like. Indeed, although some price discussions must come from the physician himself at the time that treatment options are actually being discussed, in many cases it may be preferable to invite the patient to discuss prices and other financial questions with such office personnel. The patient may be less likely to suppose that the physician's primary concern is in being paid if such matters are handled by someone other than himself. Reciprocally, if the physician sincerely invites the patient to discuss with him any economic problems that his treatment poses, the patient may perceive that the physician cares about him as a person, not just as a medical patient.

The physician might also wish to print up basic information about payment expectations, investment or incentive conflicts, and the like in a brochure to be presented to new patients.[41] Computers, too, can help to keep track of important information about prices of products and services, and can make that information quickly and easily available to the physician and his business staff. Electronic claims processing can likewise help to expedite financial management.

Other forms of practical assistance in economic disclosure and advocacy can be found on a broader level. Two are particularly important. From the proliferation of third-party payers, each with its own, often idiosyncratic, forms of cost containment, there has emerged an extraordinary and confusing array of requirements that must be satisfied before providers or patients can be reimbursed.[42] This "hassle factor" is now the target of intense critical scrutiny as physicians, organizations, and even the Federal government attempt to reduce the bureaucratic red tape that sometimes interferes considerably with patient care. Clearly, needless hassles should be eliminated. They consume enormous amounts of time that should otherwise be spent on patient care, and they extinguish much of the joy that many physicians once found in their profession.

The other form of broader practical assistance should be monetary. Careful conversation with patients takes time, and physicians' time is valuable. They should be paid for important counseling services. This point is already partly recognized as the Federal Medicare program begins to reimburse physicians on a relative value scale, wherein cognitive services are to be better paid, with correspondingly less emphasis on top-dollar compensation for procedural services.[43] It is to be hoped that the health care financing system will devote more systematic attention to the value of physician–patient conversations and will compensate physicians better for their new duties of economic advocacy and economic advising.

Fourth and finally, the physician should take appropriate steps to ensure that the economic circumstances that he discloses to patients are themselves morally acceptable. He should not merely disclose his fees, but should actually keep them reasonable. As one observer has noted, "it seems quite likely that only when physicians take their own incomes seriously as an ethical problem will they be able to regain a sense of trust in the public forum."[44] And physicians should take care that the incentive schemes and investments to which they agree do not create morally untenable conflicts. While the physician cannot entirely avoid conflicts of interest and of obligation, he can and should do his best to ameliorate them wherever possible. In this sense the awkwardness of economic disclosures can actually be useful. If the physician cannot think of any way to explain or justify a particular fee structure or incentive arrangement to his patient, then perhaps the fee or incentive itself needs to be reconsidered.[45] Let us, then, look more closely at the physician's obligations regarding his affiliations with health care institutions.

Institutional Arrangements

Physicians must consider institutional arrangements on two levels: they must examine closely the particular payer or provider institutions with which they choose to be personally affiliated, and they must think about the broader institutions by which health care is delivered in society.

Individual physicians can be associated with institutions as employees, as independent contractors, or as entrepreneurial investors. As employees or independent contractors, physicians are particularly susceptible to external controls on their decision making, or to incentive schemes designed to influence their decisions. As investors, physicians can control their decisions and their resources as they wish, but at the cost of directly creating a conflict between their interests and their patients'. In any case, institutions are now systematically and intimately interposed in physicians' relationships with their patients.

Problems can arise in this context, partly because in most cases the physician has made a voluntary commitment to the institution, and the institution has every right to expect his cooperation with important institutional goals such as the nasty necessity of cost containment. He must not renege without compelling cause.

Further problems arise because physicians and organizations can have very different needs and goals. Organizations have a high need for predictability and for close coordination and integration among their services and departments. They serve broad goals of public service and organizational effectiveness, and are generally accountable to a broader public rather than to any particular individual. Physicians, in contrast, focus on the narrower needs of individual patients. They must have the freedom to operate within the considerable uncertainties of the clinical setting, and traditionally they are professionally accountable almost exclusively to the particular patients they serve.[46] Because their goals and operations are thus so disparate, it should come as no surprise that organizations occasionally place physicians under incentives that conflict with physicians' professional goals to serve patients' interests. How, then, should physicians arrange their institutional obligations in order to ensure a minimum of interference with their obligations to patients?

As a prospective employee or independent contractor, the physician must scrutinize closely the proposed terms of any institutional relationship. He must look carefully, for example, to discern just what sort of salary contingencies or bonus payments might be tied to particular patient care decisions; what hidden cost containment mechanisms might eventually influence his behavior; what restrictions are placed on referrals; what limits utilization reviewers can place on his decisions; and what corporate definitions and expectations of productivity will be applied to his work.[47] In the process, the physician must insist that the institution provide complete and accurate information—an economic full disclosure or informed consent for the physician himself—before he agrees to any contract.[48] He is also well advised to enlist competent counsel to examine a prospective contract before signing.[49]

As he examines any proposed incentive arrangement, the physician should keep several important considerations in mind. Though every compensation system will have its adverse incentives,[50] some arrangements are morally more dubious than others. First, the connection between the incentives and individual patient care decisions should be as remote as possible (unless, of course, the incentives are designed to enhance the patient's interests, as for example to reward improvements in quality of care[51]). Incentives that reward groups for overall performance have far less impact on individual patient care decisions than those rewarding the individual physician for making particular preferred decisions, or even rewarding the individual for his own overall (e.g., year-end) performance.[52] Beyond this, incentives' size should be kept as small as possible. They should be designed to prompt the physician to consider costs appropriately—to remind him pointedly that economics really does matter—but not to distort his reasoning. A well-designed incentive should prompt the physician to consider more carefully what he does with clinical uncertainties and borderline options; it should not induce or even incline him to forgo what he believes is clearly in the patient's interest.[53]

Physicians can also participate actively in institutions' management and medical governance. Studies have shown that where physicians actively help hospitals to decide, for example, on equipment purchases, scheduling of patient care, treatment protocols, coordination of services, and the like, quality of care can improve while costs actually go down.[54] Other observers, in the same vein, argue that physicians should not only be active but also as independent as possible in their management roles.[55]

Physicians as investors can likewise take care to minimize conflicts of interest and maximize their capacity to serve patients' welfare. They should closely supervise, if not actively manage, their purchased facilities in order to ensure quality of care and fairness of fees. They may establish procedures to waive charges for indigent patients. Where the physician is likely to refer his own patients to his investment facility, he can ameliorate conflicts of interest in a variety of ways, as through careful disclosure to both patients and payers; informing the patient about alternative facilities; basing returns on the size of investment rather than on the number of referrals; engaging independent utilization review; and inviting nonphysicians to invest.[56]

Physicians also have some responsibility to influence institutional arrangements on a broader level. We noted in Chapter 5 that, as those closest not only to patients' needs but also to various institutions' failures in meeting those needs, physicians are especially prepared to inform government and corporate policy makers about the specific ways in which health care institutions can be improved.[57]

With conscientiousness and care, physicians should be able to forge institutional relationships that permit them to honor their most basic commitments to serve their patients. "The question is not to find a set of incentives that is beyond criticism, but to seek arrangements that encourage the physician to function as a professional, in the highest sense of the term."[58]

THE LIMITS OF FIDELITY

Even the simplistic traditional view of fidelity that we have rejected had its caveats. The physician has never been expected to accept literally every patient who asks for care; he is not expected to forgo all personal life, relaxation, and monetary reward; he is not required to expose himself to virtually suicidal risks in order to treat his patients, particularly where there is very little chance that his efforts will alter the patient's course. Such care during times of plague is commonly considered medical heroism.[59]

Still, a stout preeminence of patient interests over physician interests has been morally *de rigueur*. And it has been relatively easy to fulfill. In days of lavish insurance, physicians' interests largely coincided with patients'. For the most part, the physician needed only to forgo the temptation to garner extra fees by performing excessive interventions. It should be clear by now that this comfortable situation has changed dramatically as physicians are routinely placed in conflicts of interest and often must pay a substantial price if they wish to be their patients' best advocate. We must therefore consider more carefully than ever just what level of dedication is morally required and, conversely, the limits of fidelity—what is above and beyond the call of duty.

We can look for clues in the emerging literature on physicians' obligations to care for patients with AIDS or other deadly diseases, for here, too, we seek an appropriate balance between risk to the physician and benefit to the patient.[60] Three broad factors seem particularly important.

First, the likelihood and magnitude of the patient's need and expected benefit must be considered. Where administrators pressure an emergency room physician to dump onto a public hospital an unstable, indigent patient with a serious gunshot wound, that patient could suffer serious impairment, exacerbation of illness, or even death. In contrast, a patient with a relatively uncomplicated viral respiratory infection might be transferred with considerably less risk of harm. Clearly, the more serious and urgent the patient's need, the more serious and urgent is the physician's obligation try to meet that need.

Second, we must consider the nature and magnitude of the physician's prospective sacrifice. There are interesting differences between the physical risks of treating AIDS and the fiscal and professional risks the physician incurs in pursuing health care resources for his patients. A physical risk is ordinarily confined to each instance of hazardous patient care. Once the invasive procedure is finished, or once the patient has left the office or is discharged from the hospital, the physician's risk is gone.

In contrast, economic risks are usually cumulative. Rarely will one decision to prolong a patient's hospital stay result in administrative pressures; neither will just one decision to refer a patient for specialist consultation within an HMO substantially alter one's year-end income. Yet through case after case, the pressures on the physician to meet economic goals can be substantial. In a sense, the difference is like that between commodity scarcity and fiscal scarcity. Whereas the former is episodic, the latter is chronic and permeates all one's decisions. In point of fact, some physicians consider these new resource burdens to be considerably more onerous than physical risks. One internist, interviewing a number of colleagues, indicated that they "all said that they vastly preferred caring for patients with any disease [including AIDS] to struggles with insurance companies."[61] The financial and professional sacrifices of the new economics, though incremental, can be substantial.

In each case it is important to inquire, as accurately as possible, just what price the physician really is likely to pay for that particular proposed pursuit of patient benefit. Empty speculation or knee-jerk panic will not suffice. How annoyed, really, will the hospital administrator be if I keep Mr. Smith here another day and order another round of lab studies? Can't I negotiate reasonably with him if he challenges me? How long will it actually take to complete the required phone calls to secure utilization approval for Mrs. Jones' elective surgery? Are there more efficient ways to discharge such responsibilities?

Because of the cumulative character of the physician's sacrifices, however, it is also important to consider what overall penalty he stands to incur if he makes similar resource decisions in similar cases. Even though one might make extra demands on resources in any one case without paying a serious penalty, one cannot do so as a rule without eventually paying the price. One may be able to run another round of lab tests specifically for Mr. Smith, but if nearly all one's patients use markedly more resources than is average for other patients at this hospital, then one will likely incur the eventual wrath of the administration.

Admittedly, realistic predictions of the physician's sacrifices may be difficult to make. And yet careful thought and close observation of the institutional payers and providers with whom one actually works can at least help the individual physician to construct increasingly factual, and less speculative, estimates of the consequences he may incur for vigorous patient advocacy.

Third, the physician needs to consider competing obligations. Other patients, institutional commitments, and fellow health care workers can all warrant concern. For example, the physician who refuses to help contain costs at a financially pressed hospital may be unfairly shifting onto his colleagues the moral as well as economic burdens of helping to keep the hospital solvent.[62] He who routinely orders his laboratory tests to be run "stat" (immediately) can overburden the laboratory and thereby cause delays for other physicians who need to order lab tests for their patients.

Ratzan and Schneiderman offer a useful broad-spectrum concept to summarize these three factors. The physician, they suggest, owes his patient a "critical minimum equivalent effort."[63] "Critical minimum" refers to that societally expected "reasonable expenditure of a physician's skill and knowledge to alleviate pain, cure illness, and support function." While a physician is not expected to risk virtually certain suicide in the care of a patient, it is equally clear that he should be willing to risk more than the dirtying of his dinner clothes.

The concept of "equivalent effort," while acknowledging that each patient is different, suggests that the physician should be willing to incur comparable levels of risk or inconvenience in comparable situations.[64] In a way, this notion is rather like the rule of thumb introduced in the last chapter. Just as the physician should only press resources as far as he can justify others' pressing them in similar ways for similar reasons, the reasonable limits on his efforts for any particular patient are determined by looking at the total level of effort that he would devote if he treated all his patients in the same way. It is reasonable to expect that he make phone calls to utilization reviewers, for example, and that he make some effort to challenge inappropriate denials of payment authorization. No physician, however, could afford routinely to spend literally hours in this effort for each and every patient.

Note also, that the limits of the physician's advocacy obligations also depend on the particular requirements set out for each obligation. In fulfilling insurance requirements, for example, the physician's obligation is basically to respond to a specific request, such as to make a phone call, to sign a claim form, to explain the medical necessity of the patient's care. Where repeated efforts to phone the UR office yield only a series of busy signals or a string of thirty-minute on-hold waits, the physician may be justified to inform the patient of the problem and encourage him to pursue a solution. It is the patient who owes payment to the physician, after all, and if his chosen payer somehow precludes the physician from fulfilling its own requirements, the patient has a responsibility to help investigate the matter. In other cases the physician may be required to do more work if his initial effort was inadequate. If his justification of medical necessity was too cursory or his supplemental documentation inadequate, an insurer may be entirely justified in requesting him to fulfill its procedures better.

From a purely prudential viewpoint, it may be wise for physicians to document the ways in which health care's economic arrangements make patient care more difficult or require excessive effort. One can document UR phone calls, for instance, noting especially those instances in which multiple calls are required for a single proposed intervention, or those UR companies that seem more often to obstruct care than to establish economic legitimacy. The physician might also consider charging a fee for excessive time spent on insurance requirements or, collectively, encouraging his hospital to pay a physician colleague to undertake some of the more routine tasks of utilization review.[65] With systematic data and a bit of inventiveness, physicians may be able actually to help improve the structure of health care delivery and, thereby, in the long run to reduce needless distractions from patient care.

In the final analysis, we cannot expect precise or tidy formulae. In ethics, as in medicine, "cookbooks" are at best guidelines that cannot supplant a sensitivity to the details of the case. Here, our guiding concept is reasonableness. We ask the physician for serious dedication, but cannot demand unreasonable personal sacrifice. And yet the concept of reasonableness is admittedly vague: "Every complaint that a doctor didn't make a house call in an ice storm represents an unresolved difference of opinion about what constitutes a reasonable sacrifice."[66]

In spite of its pivotal importance, there does not appear to be any way of answering this question in the abstract. The most that can be said here, I think, is that gauging the precise threshold between strict duty and supererogation will always be a matter of practical judgment strongly influenced by socially and historically determined views of what counts as a 'reasonable' risk. Procedurally, this requires an ongoing dialogue between professionals on the firing line and the rest of society.[67]

NOTES

1. This distinction is offered by Jennings, Callahan, and Caplan, 1988, p. 10, to describe the differences in the ways we view acute versus chronic illness. The distinction is useful also when applied to physicians' new relationship to resources.

2. Ratzan and Schneiderman, 1988; Arras, 1988; Emanuel, 1988; Zuger and Miles, 1987; Miller, 1983.

3. Pellegrino and Thomasma, 1981; see also Zuger and Miles, 1987, p. 1927; Hiatt, 1987, pp. 38–40.

4. Zuger and Miles, 1987, p. 1927; Cassell, 1986, p. 201 ff.; H. Brody, 1987, p. 16; Daniels, 1987.

5. Daniels, 1987, p. 71; Daniels, 1986, p. 1382.

6. Shepherd, 1981, p. 326.

7. Schaber and Rohwer, 1984; Morreim, 1991.

8. Miller, 1983, p. 164.

9. Holder, 1978, p. 255; Veatch, 1983, p. 144 ff.; *Salgo v. Stanford*, 1957; *Natanson v. Kline*, 1960; *Canterbury v. Spence*, 1972; *Cobbs v. Grant*, 1972.

10. *Cobbs v. Grant*, 1972, p. 9.

11. Rie and Engelhardt, 1989.

12. Butler and Haislmaier, 1989, pp. 6–28, 57; Eddy, 1990(a), p. 1165.

13. Eddy, 1990(a), p. 1165.

14. See discussion in Chapter 3.

15. Alderman, 1989, p. 126, n. 90; Wennberg, 1990.

16. Hippocrates, cited in Lachs, Sindelar, and Horwitz, 1990, p. 1600.

17. Johns and Fortuin, 1988.

18. Alderman, 1989, p. 129.

19. Ibid., 1989, p. 129 ff.

20. Ibid., p. 129; Merken, 1989.

21. Grumet, 1989. Where patients are unfairly denied coverage to which they thought they were entitled, they do have some legal recourse through civil lawsuits. And in such suits they do have some advantages, since courts tend to interpret insurers' policy ambiguities in favor of the insured. *Sarchett v. Blue Shield of California*, 1987; Abraham, 1981. The patient's real need in the decision-making context, however, is for early and accurate information about coverage. This need is hardly satisfied by the prospect of a costly, even if successful, lawsuit to avenge failures of disclosure or owed payments.

22. Bock, 1988.

23. Astrachan and Astrachan, 1989, p. 1511; Hillman, 1990, p. 892.

24. Kellermann and Ackerman, 1988, p. 643.

25. Stern, 1983; Scovern, 1988; Povar and Moreno, 1988; Grumet, 1989.

26. In one case Sharon Bush, a subscriber in a Michigan HMO, presented to her primary physician with vaginal bleeding unrelated to menstruation.

Without performing a Pap smear to check for cervical cancer, Dr. Paul Dake empirically prescribed antibiotics for a presumed infection. Several months later when the problem had not yet resolved, Dake referred Bush to a gynecologist within the HMO. Because Dake had not requested it, the gynecologist did not perform a Pap test either, but instead prescribed (different) antibiotics, again for a presumed infection. When the problem persisted several months more, Bush sought care outside the HMO, whereupon she was diagnosed with cervical cancer. Bush sued both physicians and the HMO, not only on the ground that her care fell below medical standards, but because the HMOs incentive system encouraged such substandard practices and because the system was not disclosed to her. Had she known of it, she argued, she would have been far more skeptical of the medical advice she received. The case was eventually settled out of court under terms that were not disclosed. See Geyelin, 1990; Meyer, 1987(b); Meyer, 1989(a); Stern, 1983; Alderman, 1989; Morreim, 1990(c).

27. Morreim, 1989(a).
28. Morreim, 1987; Morreim, 1989(c).
29. Furrow, 1986.
30. Morreim, 1986(b).
31. Morreim, 1987.
32. Hall, 1989; Morreim, 1989(c).
33. Ore. Rev. Stat. Ann. 414.720 *et. seq.*, 1989.
34. Ore. Rev. Stat. Ann. 414.725, Section 6 (7).
35. Ore. Rev. Stat. Ann. 414.745, Section 10.
36. Morreim, 1987; Morreim, 1989(c).
37. The Oregon provisions discussed just above could actually be encompassed within this divided standard of care. On this view, we would say that the state has set the standard of resource use for its own Medicaid citizens and that, although that standard might be below that received by some other citizens (particularly during times of a shortfall in state funds), it would still serve as the resource baseline for this particular group of people. The physician who delivers that particular SRU then would not be held liable simply because it is less than other SRUs.
38. *Wickline v. State of California*, 1986.
39. Butler, 1985, p. 364.
40. See Mechanic, 1986, pp. 53–54, for a discussion of ways in which physicians can help patients to adjust their expectations.
41. Such careful explanations not only honor the patient's need and right to economic information; they can actually help improve the physician's billing collections. See Berry, 1990.
42. Grumet, 1989.
43. Iglehart, 1990; Hsiao, Braun, Ynetma et al., 1988; Hsiao, Braun, Dunn et al., 1988; Hsiao et al., 1987; Lee et al., 1989; U.S. Congress, 1989, p. H–9354 ff.

44. H. Brody, 1987, p. 16.

45. For a more detailed discussion of economic disclosure, see Morreim, 1991.

46. Shortell, 1983, p. 86 ff.

47. Page, 1987(b); Hillman, 1987, p. 1747; Marcus, 1984, p. 1509; American Society of Internal Medicine, 1987; Bock, 1988; Scovern, 1988; Hillman, 1990, p. 892.

48. Engelhardt and Rie, 1988, p. 1088.

49. American Society of Internal Medicine, 1987; Sharfstein and Beigel, 1988, p. 726.

50. Institute of Medicine, 1986, p. 153.

51. Meyer, 1988.

52. Institute of Medicine, 1986, p. 162 ff.; Brock, 1986, p. 768; Hillman, 1990, p. 891.

53. Hillman, 1990.

54. Shortell, 1983, p. 90 ff; Omenn and Conrad, 1984, p. 1315; Institute of Medicine, 1986, pp. 173–79.

55. Astrachan and Astrachan, 1989.

56. Morreim, 1989(a); Todd and Horan, 1989.

57. Astrachan and Astrachan, 1989, p. 1511; Sharfstein and Beigel, 1988; Furrow, 1988; Pellegrino, 1986.

58. Institute of Medicine, 1986, p. 153.

59. Zuger and Miles, 1987, p. 1926; Ratzan and Schneiderman, 1988; Arras, 1988.

60. Arras, 1988; Emanuel, 1988; Ratzan and Schneiderman, 1988; Zuger and Miles, 1987.

61. Platt, 1989, p. 1724.

62. Morreim, 1985(a).

63. Ratzan and Schneiderman, 1988, p. 3468.

64. Ibid., p. 3468.

65. Larkin, 1990.

66. Ratzan and Schneiderman, 1988, p. 3466.

67. Arras, 1988, p. 16.

7

The New Medical Ethics of Medicine's New Economics

Probably the most important implication of medicine's economic revolution is that it forces us to reconsider not just financial arrangements, but also some long and widely held tenets of medical ethics. Initially, physicians' obligations of fidelity stemmed from patients' substantial vulnerability. Illness, impairment, ignorance, and an imbalance of power in the physician–patient relationship gave rise to strong duties of personal and professional fidelity. Since the advent of modern bioethics over the past three decades, this traditional view has been powerfully augmented by another concept, patient autonomy. Coincident with early legal cases establishing the doctrine of informed consent,[1] early bioethics literature argued vigorously against long-standing physician paternalism in favor of the view that competent patients are entitled to make their own medical decisions.[2] Whereas the older, vulnerability-based ethic of fidelity required the physician to promote the patient's benefit in whatever ways the physician thought best, autonomy-based fidelity requires the physician to promote the patient's benefit as the patient himself defines it.

AUTONOMY AS FREEDOM

Largely because of this initial concern to defeat paternalism, early bioethics literature tended to define autonomy quite exclusively in terms of freedom—both the internal freedom of the competent person to make his own choices, and his external freedom to carry those choices out. As noted by Beauchamp and Childress, autonomy is the "personal rule of the self while remaining free from both the controlling interferences by others and personal limitations, such as inadequate understanding, that prevent meaningful choice."[3] To honor this capacity for reflective choice is, after all, not only to benefit individuals and promote their happiness; it is integral to our respect for them as having unconditional moral worth.[4]

131

More recent bioethics literature has added a level of sophistication in recognizing that patients do not always come to the physician with clear minds and clear preferences. The physician does not honor autonomy simply by deferring to the first thing the patient says, taken at face value. Rather, he has a duty to help patients to overcome the medical and emotional impediments to sound decision-making and thereby to ascertain more fully what they want. Still, the emphasis remains on maximizing and respecting the patient's freedom to do whatever he (really) wants.[5]

Note, this emphasis on autonomy as personal freedom can be traced to a fundamental ethic within Western, and particularly American, society in which moral analysis in general is directed primarily toward individuals and their rights of independence, privacy, self-reliance, and freedom from outside intervention.[6] It is an ethic reflected in an early flag of the American republic, featuring a serpent and the legend, "Don't tread on me."

This heavy concentration on autonomy-as-freedom has had important implications for our most prevalent ethical descriptions of the physician–patient relationship. The patient's interests are of course paramount, as required already under the vulnerability-based view. But now the patient himself defines his own well-being and decides how best to pursue it.

This ethic, in turn, has been reflected in a number of specific arrangements. Economically, as we have seen, many observers have thought it imperative to insulate patients from worries about costs at the time of medical decision-making. To limit his choices on economic grounds is, after all, to constrain his freedom, which in turn is seen in this view to violate his autonomy. While it is roundly agreed that respect for autonomy would forbid the physician to inflict unwanted care upon a hopelessly ill patient,[7] reciprocally it would equally affront autonomy to deny any medically acceptable intervention, even sophisticated intensive care, to the patient or family who says "do everything."[8]

This pattern of economic insulation persists even throughout many of the newest cost containment arrangements. Though patients of course are now expected to pay higher cost-sharing, this is often quite limited; most incentive arrangements are directed toward physicians. The HMO physician, not the patient, has a higher year-end income if he is frugal about ordering tests and consults; the surgeon, not the patient, wins bonus money if the patient is discharged from the hospital a day or two early. Few incentives are aimed at patients, and those that are have come under intense scrutiny.[9] Although these economic arrangements are, of course, the product of other factors as well, nevertheless our emphasis on patients' freedom to do as they please looms large.

Our moral expectations of physicians have similarly been shaped by this heavy emphasis on autonomy-as-freedom. We expect the physician to help the patient make choices and, although he must be ready to provide information, answer questions, and assist the patient, he must not impose his own preferences. He is expected, too, to protect the patient against undue influences, whether others' or his own. The physician must offer "only the highest quality of medical care to each individual . . . must refuse to buckle to shameful government pressures;"[10] he must "not allow consideration of his economic or career interests to influence his treatment of his patient."[11] Legally, too, physicians have been expected to exhibit the undivided loyalty expected of all fiduciaries,[12] and to ensure that the care they deliver meets the prevailing standard, regardless of the patient's financial circumstances.[13]

Our notion of autonomy-as-freedom has even suggested that patients should be insulated from social factors that might impinge on their decisions in medically unfavorable ways. If a patient wants to leave the hospital earlier than is medically advisable in order to return to his job, he might well be accused of denial, or of failing to appreciate the importance of his health. If a patient states that he does not want heroic life-saving interventions because he does not want to drain his family's resources, at least some suspicion may arise that his family are somehow pressuring him inappropriately.[14] Where a newborn is seriously impaired, many observers would consider it morally highly suspect even to consider the burdens that his handicapped life will pose for his family.[15] Or if a researcher is offering to pay his subjects too much, he might be accused of attempting to sway those subjects to think more than they should about the money and not enough about their best medical interests.[16] Indeed, wherever the patient expresses serious concern about matters other than his own best medical interests, one is likely to find some commentator expressing the fear that something is wrong, since the patient is failing to give his health top priority.

The net result of much of the bioethics literature's longstanding emphasis on patient autonomy is a markedly atomistic, insular picture in which the physician is expected to attend almost exclusively to his patient,[17] and in which all others, whether courts, risk managers, society at large, insurers, or other economic agents, are identified as "intruders."[18] Because all of them may try in various ways to limit patients' medical options or to influence patients' or physicians' choices, these assorted third parties are regarded as unwelcome invaders into an otherwise sacrosanct relationship.

Unfortunately, the view of autonomy on which this conception of the physician–patient relationship is based, together with all its moral, economic, legal, and social implications, is essentially untenable. To view human autonomy exclusively or even primarily as a matter of promoting human freedom is to miss the pivotal moral feature of autonomy: responsibility.

AUTONOMY AS RESPONSIBILITY

Virtually any sentient creature might be said to benefit from some measure of freedom and noninterference, but for persons the moral significance of freedom is much different. What makes a competent human being morally distinctive is not just some bare capacity to choose A over B or to enact such choices. Rather, our moral distinctiveness is our capacity to reflect on our choices and on the values and beliefs behind them and, in so doing, to engage in self-determination at the deepest level. By making such evaluations we literally determine what sort of self we are. We decide what sort of person we want to be, what sort of life we wish to live, and we act accordingly in the myriad small and large choices that we face. In so doing, we assert a special authorship over our decisions and actions. We say that they are ours in the most profound sense—not that they simply happened to occur in our presence or with the involvement of our bodies, but that these decisions and actions are ours by deliberate choice.

This personal ownership makes one morally an agent, a doer, not merely a passive receiver of events. And it renders one personally, morally accountable for his conduct in a way that could not possibly be ascribed to a being who had no such authorship. Such an agent is capable of bearing praise and blame, and of engaging in genuine moral discourse.[19]

It is this capacity to be an agent, to bear responsibility for decisions and actions that are truly one's own, that renders a person worthy of moral respect, dignity, as beyond merely considerate treatment. On this account, then, freedom is not the central focus of moral autonomy, but rather a prerequisite. One can only be a morally special, responsible agent if and when he has the freedom truly to be his own person, to make his own choices and claim the necessary authorship over them. We do not, after all, blame or praise people for their actions if they could not have done other than as they did. And we do not hold special respect for a being who cannot be other than as he is and who cannot own up to his values, choices, and actions.

The bioethics literature's nearly exclusive (almost obsessive) preoccupation with freedom, and its pervasive failure to ascribe responsibility to patients,[20] has had a profound impact on our most common conceptions of the physician–patient relationship. On the one hand, we have seen inordinately great responsibilities ascribed to physicians and other providers in order to shield patients from the slightest impingement on their freedom. On the other hand, a concomitant unwillingness to ascribe responsibilities to patients has ill-served them at least as much. We will look at both these consequences.

Consider first the role of the physician. To the extent that we think patients must have virtually unfettered freedom while bearing few if any responsibilities, we have reciprocally asked physicians to fill the void by assuming extra responsibility. We have asked not only that the physician permit the patient to make decisions if the patient wishes to, but we have conversely assumed that if the patient does not so desire, then the physician must make the decisions for him.[21] That is, the patient must be free not just to decide what he wants to do, but even to decide whether he wants to decide, and whether he wants to hear information relevant to such a decision. Many commentators accept almost without question the putative right of the patient to say "Don't bother me with the details, doc—you just decide what to do."[22] By expecting the physician to go along with such a request, we are asking him not only to be responsible for his own decisions as a physician, but to take responsibility as well for important choices in the patient's life. He must make not only the relevant medical decisions, such as which diagnosis is most likely to be correct, but also the relevant value choices, such as the decision whether the benefits of a surgical procedure are worth the risks of permanent injury or even death.

The presumption goes even further. While many physicians and bioethicists readily warrant that the patient "must be *allowed* to share in the medical decision-making process if he wishes to do so,"[23] they equally insist the physician must never force him to do so, particularly where very difficult decisions must be made. In intensive care units it is common for physicians to emphasize to each another that they must not require the patient or family to decide whether to withdraw life support since, after all, the family could face terrible guilt afterwards.[24] While the patient or family is entirely free to refuse the physician's plan, so the reasoning goes, the physician is morally obligated to assume the overall responsibility.[25] He thus supposes that he is obligated to "prophylax" families for guilt by taking the decision, and with it all the guilt, upon himself. To put the matter more starkly: while we castigate the physician wherever he would purport to "play God,"[26] we nevertheless require him to "play Christ."

Yet surely this view about physicians' responsibilities is unfounded. Why, we must inquire, must the physician make decisions for a competent patient or family member, simply because the questions are difficult or their consequences sad, or because the patient or surrogate does not happen to want to shoulder the responsibility himself? We can appreciate the oddness of this presumption even more forcefully by considering one of the few areas of medical practice where it does not prevail: genetic counseling. The woman who has just learned that her three-month-old fetus has a serious genetic disorder may face a sad and difficult decision about whether to terminate her pregnancy. And yet, if she implores her physician, "I just don't know what to do—you decide," surely no serious geneticist would respond by saying, "All right. I've decided you're going to have an abortion. We'll do it tomorrow at two o'clock." Rather, he would respond that this just isn't the sort of decision that he can or should make.[27] Serious values are at stake, of an obviously nonmedical nature.

The example is poignant for its contrast value, because physicians routinely make just such value decisions in other contexts. If a patient with cancer says, "You decide, doctor, whether I should have surgery, radiation, or chemotherapy," many physicians will make such a decision without hesitation, even though equally personal values—values such as the appropriate balance between length of life and quality of life—are at stake.[28]

If our conception of autonomy-*sans*-responsibility places undue burdens on physicians, its implications for patients are at least as serious. On the most basic level, the failure to treat a competent patient as being responsible to make his own decisions and be accountable for them is a profound moral insult. It is to presume that he is not fully a moral agent, that he is something less than the capable adult that physicians and other citizens are, and that he must be treated at least partly as a child.

This presumption that patients are not fully responsible agents actually has had important ramifications. First, let us recall that third-party reimbursements were for many years structured to insulate the patient from worrying about costs at the time of decision-making. In so doing, they also carried a serious potential for undercutting the patient's active participation in decision-making or even his interest in hearing the medical information that might be relevant to his decision. Where the patient pays nothing for the costly diagnostic test, he may be far less inclined to inquire closely about whether it is really worth undertaking, even from a purely medical standpoint.[29] If his physician thinks it ought to be done, and it won't cost him a cent, then why waste time on the details?

At the same time, where patients exhibit little direct interest in learning about the details of their medical situation and options, or in assuming responsibility for making their own decisions, it becomes ever easier for physicians to regard them as childlike, treat them accordingly, and ultimately to foster a self-fulfilling prophecy of infantile behavior.[30]

Further, the more our concept of autonomy ignores the central element of moral responsibility, the easier it becomes to medicalize problematic behavior, reclassifying as a disease many kinds of conduct that would otherwise be regarded as offensive, nasty, lazy, obnoxious, or downright evil. To be ill, after all, is to have no immediate responsibility for one's condition.[31]

Such medicalization raises important issues. On the one hand, reclassifying a behavior from offense to disease permits us to offer help without condemnation. We may entice the drug abuser, the excessive gambler, or even the profligate spender to seek help, if he knows that we will not chastise him when he comes to us. One does not, after all, praise or blame those conditions for which the individual is not responsible. On the other hand, to declare a person's conduct to be the product of disease rather than free choice is to presuppose that that person is less than a full moral agent. Thereby, it is to presuppose that he is not entitled to the full measure of dignity and respect reserved only for those who are moral agents. He will receive not the praise or blame of those who fully own their acts, but rather the benevolent hand that we extend to the infantile or infirm.[32] Callahan expresses the problem well:

> [M]atters get out of hand when all physical, mental and communal disorders are put under the heading of 'sickness', and all sufferers (all of us, in the end) placed in the blameless 'sick role'. Not only are the concepts of 'sickness' and 'illness' drained of all content, it also becomes impossible to ascribe any freedom or responsibility to those caught up in the throes of illness. The whole world is sick, and no one is responsible any longer for anything. That is determinism gone mad . . .[33]

Finally, the notion of autonomy-*sans*-responsibility leads to an extraordinarily atomistic view not only of the physician–patient relationship, but of patients and their social selves.[34] We have already noted that where a physician dares to consider the social or economic costs of the care he renders to his patient, he is rather likely to be accused of disloyalty. And where a patient worries about the effect that his illness will have on his family or his job, or even about its costs to his insurer, someone will probably question his competence or others' influence. Such an atomistic isolationism is unfortunate. However much we may agree that the individual person is a morally important unit, human beings and human morality are intensely social. Moral rights and wrongs concern the ways in which people treat one another, and indeed an individual's sense of his own self is defined at least partly by his place in his community. Inasmuch as traditional bioethics literature focuses on autonomy as individual freedom, to the neglect of responsibility, it isolates the physician–patient relationship from the world and the society in which health and human functioning have their purpose. If such atomism has been the case hitherto, it is now time to return health and healing to its broader social context.

THE NEW MEDICAL ETHICS

Perhaps the most positive consequence of medicine's economic revolution is that it forces us not only to reevaluate our economic arrangements, but to examine basic ideas about medical ethics that should have been reconsidered long ago, quite apart from any connection with economics. We have already seen that a thin and inadequate concept of autonomy-as-freedom has undergirded much of modern bio-ethics. It is time now to replace the more simplistic ideals of the past with an enhanced appreciation of complexity, and substantially to revise the roles that we have assigned to both patients and physicians.

The complexity of medicine's new economics should by now be obvious. Where earlier we could speak of a basically dyadic relationship between physician and patient, funded by silent partners, we must now acknowledge an enormous number of players in complex concatenations of relationships. While physicians still have the authority to decide which interventions to identify for patients' consideration and the power to open the door to any intervention requiring a medical prescription, other parties now control crucial elements in health care. Insurers, governments, private corporations, and institutional providers now generally determine which technologies will be developed, and how quickly; which technologies will be locally available, and to whom; what level of funding will be available for which interventions for what kinds of patients; what sorts of incentives will limit and direct physicians' and patients' choices; which sorts of medical practice will, and will not, be attractive for physicians to enter; and what sorts of health care will, and will not, be attractive for patients to accept.[35] These parties are not intruders[36] into the physician–patient relationship. In many ways, they make that relationship possible. The wisest, most skilled physician can do little if he has no tools. Those tools are created, and their use made financially available, by the many "intruders" who now play such a prominent role in health care. Within this world of new complexity, we may now consider the respective roles of patients and physicians.

Patients

We begin with patients. In matters of health, and of health care, it is time to expect competent[37] patients to assume substantially greater responsibility. In the first place, they should generally make their own decisions. Not only is the patient entitled to decide these issues that affect his life so fundamentally; he has a presumptive obligation to do so.

This obligation is best seen as an *in rem* duty, that is, a duty owed to all.[38] It is a justice-based obligation of every agent to "carry his own weight" in the moral community. One must not only fulfill the specific responsibilities that are expected of all moral agents—duties such as keeping one's promises—but should also refrain from imposing unfair burdens on others. Here, it means that each person has at least a *prima facie* responsibility to make his own life decisions and not presumptively to impose on someone else the burden of making them. The bare fact that a decision is difficult or sad does not entail, *ipso facto*, that others must therefore make it for him and bear its consequences. Those others, after all, have difficult choices of their own.[39]

To expect anything less of a patient is to regard him as something less than a real moral agent. It is to demean, not honor, his autonomy. Thus, we must reject the idea that the patient should be shielded from making difficult decisions, or that the physician's job description somehow automatically requires him to shoulder the patient's decision-making responsibility.

There are some important caveats. First, not all patients are competent to assume such responsibility. Health care concerns disease and disability, after all, and these can be associated with a range of impairments in one's capacity to make his own decisions.[40]

However, even this fact does not warrant a presumption that the physician must automatically step into the breach. Although it is common to think of the patient as being hopelessly vulnerable in the medical setting, in many cases this isn't true. Because bioethicists do much of their work in tertiary care teaching hospitals, it is easy for them to slip into the view that most medical decisions concern people who are desperately ill. In fact, however, most encounters between physician and patient are for such mundane matters as routine physical examinations and screening tests, short-term management of self-limiting illnesses or minor accidents, and long-term care of chronic illnesses such as hypertension, diabetes, or arthritis.[41] To suppose that such patients' competence typically is seriously impaired is surely to underestimate their autonomy and, thereby, their capacity to be responsible for their own choices and consequences.

Even clear incompetence does not entail that the physician must assume responsibility for the patient's decisions. In most cases the patient will have someone available to serve as a surrogate decision maker. Indeed, competent persons arguably have some obligation to consider whom they would like to invest with decision-making authority when they are unable themselves to fulfill this responsibility. And where a surrogate is available, we can expect that person to carry out the decisional responsibilities the patient would otherwise have.

Where the patient has only a partial impairment of his capacity, he can still be involved in decision-making and, to that degree, can be expected to be accountable. To whatever extent someone has the capacity to make his own decisions—to merit the freedom from paternalist intrusion that standard bioethics literature insists on so vigorously—then to that extent he is also capable of bearing responsibility for his choices. Reciprocally, if we cannot rightly hold a person accountable for the content and consequences of his decisions, then to that extent we have, implicitly at least, determined that he is not fully a rational agent and might be subject to justifiable paternalism.[42]

To argue that the patient has presumptive responsibility to make his own health care decisions does not preclude that patient from explicitly asking the physician to make medical decisions on the patient's behalf, or that physician from freely agreeing to do so. There are many contexts in which fully autonomous individuals can convey to someone else a power of agency over certain affairs, as for example where one gives someone power of attorney over financial affairs.[43] However, such an agency role must be openly agreed to by both physician and patient, not presumed to be somehow built into the physician's job description.

The patient's obligation to make his own decisions includes not just medical choices, but also other important matters such as health care coverage.[44] It has now become important for patients to participate much more actively in choosing the plans by which their health care will be financed and delivered, for several reasons. First, it is probably impossible to contain exploding health care costs, while assuring access and quality of care, without enlisting the active cooperation of the people these plans serve. Arguably, current health care finance structures, both in the U.S. and in countries where health care is more socialized, are all encountering financial difficulties for the same reason—namely, their failure to motivate patients to insist on both value and economy.[45] As noted by Eddy[46] and other commentators, a fundamental flaw in contemporary health care systems is a severance of the usual connection between costs and value in the marketplace, wherein the person who determines the value of a good or service also pays its cost. Where one party spends and someone else pays, the inevitable result is a serious distortion of both value and cost. Without patients' involvement on both sides of the equation, this distortion probably can never be corrected.

Further, to the extent that we endorse a divided standard of care—morally, legally, or both—we thereby embrace a joint participation in establishing the standard of resource use. Since it is the patient whose life and resources are most affected by such resource standards, he should be more than a numb recipient of others' rationing decisions, but rather should be an active participant in setting the standards by which his care will be delivered. Arguably, to fail to involve patients in this way is to disrespect their autonomy, for it is to impose important economic trade-offs on them, the ultimate payers for care, without systematically incorporating their views.

Reciprocally, to involve patients more closely in choosing their health plans is probably the most acceptable way to bring rationing into the clinical setting. Throughout our lives we make trade-offs among the things we value, because everything we buy comes at the opportunity cost of foreclosing whatever we might instead have selected. To hold a competent adult to the consequences of his own trade-off decisions, even where this means informing him that he is not free to pursue certain options that he himself foreclosed, does not offend his autonomy. It honors his autonomy by respecting the choices he made for his "larger life"—not just the part of him that needs medical care.[47] If someone who has chosen a minimal health plan (e.g., to save money for skiing trips) subsequently needs the costly care that he earlier rejected, we may feel compassion for him. We may even wish charitably to help him, but we have not wronged him if we refuse, because his choice was made knowingly and rationally.[48] The physician who refrains from offering some intervention in this setting does not violate his obligations of fidelity, then, but rather is honoring the patient's own values and choices.

Note, this argument for increased patient choice among health care plans is not an argument that we must expand patients' freedom, on the ground that we somehow offend autonomy if we do not maximize people's options. Rather, the argument is that we cannot hold the patient responsible if he has not genuinely made his own decisions.

To some extent we are already seeing increased patient participation in selecting health plans. Many corporations, for example, invite employees to choose among designated health maintenance organizations, standard indemnity plans, preferred provider arrangements, or some "cafeteria" of other options.[49] Each of these plans features important trade-offs between the levels and kinds of service they make available—choices among particular providers, out-of-pocket costs levied on subscribers, basic premium costs, and the like. An invigorated view of patients' responsibilities in their own health and health care would require that we enhance and expand such choice-based plans on a national, not just corporate, level.[50]

The United States is currently on the threshold of major health policy decisions. Some observers argue on behalf of national funding for universal health care; some support a nationalized health service; some advocate a mixture of national and private funding with a vigorous competition among private providers.[51] However we resolve these questions, the considerations presented above argue that one feature should be prominent in any new health care system: patients should have a serious range of choices, and should have the largest possible voice over the trade-offs that are to be made among costs and care.

Several commentators have already proposed health systems that would emphasize consumer choice. Enthoven, for instance, would promote vigorous competition among provider organizations. Sponsoring organizations could be created to ensure that each competing health care plan is what it purports to be and that subscribers receive adequate and accurate information about each of their options. Such competing plans would then permit subscribers to choose their own cost-care trade-offs, and to enjoy the savings themselves where they choose a plan that is more efficient or more lean.[52] Several other commentators have offered fairly similar plans,[53] and still others have suggested a multiple-HMO approach.[54]

Whether or not we embrace Enthoven's or any other particular approach, we can at least agree that if the patient is to be a more responsible party in his own health care, he must have the range of choice and the decision authority that make such responsibility possible. Arguably, such choices can only take place within a system assuring universal access for all citizens. Someone who has no money with which to buy health care, after all, can hardly be said to have chosen the particular cost-care trade-offs that are placed on his care, if indeed he receives any. Similarly, we would probably need to insist that all plans include at least certain basic services. Such a requirement would protect patients from inadequate plans and, at least as important, protect everyone else from the "free rider" problem that arises when someone buys inadequate insurance with the expectation that, if he needs better care, everyone else will ante up and rescue him anyway.

Beyond such a minimum package,[55] personal choice could range over various kinds of services, such as dental care, home care, infertility treatments, or eyeglasses; the extent of services, such as to include or forgo extraordinary care for those in a medically hopeless condition; the range of choice among providers, as where one might agree to accept less costly nonmedical providers for specified sorts of care; the nature and extent of patient cost sharing, as where one might agree to accept higher out-of-pocket costs in exchange for lower overall premiums; or the provisions for resolving malpractice allegations, as by accepting binding arbitration or other alternatives to traditional tort remedies.[56]

The specifics of any particular national health plan need not trouble us here, for our only aim is to recommend greater patient choice over health care plans. The same reasoning could also apply to publicly insured patients. While government-sponsored health care programs are generally less generous than private ones, this does not preclude establishing options by which these patients, too, can choose whatever plan best suits their needs. Some commentators propose a voucher system, for example, to enable each beneficiary to choose among competing eligible programs.[57]

Patients should not only have more options, they must also have more information about their options. Each prospective health plan should inform potential (and of course current) subscribers as clearly as possible about the basic rationale, as well as the particular mechanics, of their plans. Unfortunately, such clear information is not always the norm. It can be difficult, if not impossible, for the average subscriber to get adequate and intelligible information about the various plans from which he is choosing. At best, most insurance policies are extraordinarily complex, and some policies actually are obtuse by design, in an attempt to minimize the insurer's payout obligations.[58] Similarly, HMOs and other institutional providers may provide little solid information about their limits on coverage and about the tradeoffs that they make between costs and care.[59]

Admittedly, it may be very difficult for health care plans to provide truly adequate information. Such plans are inevitably complicated, because health care's economics are immensely complex. And few people bring to the encounter much prior knowledge about health, health care, or health care economics. However, the challenge is not insuperable. We must not assume that patients are incapable of becoming sufficiently informed to make these choices, any more than we are entitled to assume that they are irrevocably too ignorant to make their own medical decisions. Several factors can ameliorate the problem.

For one thing, decisions about health care plans, unlike urgent decisions about medical treatment at a time of illness, can be made when one is healthy and fully in possession of his usual capacities for learning, reflecting, and careful decision-making. Further, better ways for conveying information can surely be devised. Corporations' benefits departments, for example, can develop improved ways of educating employees about their health care options. Physicians also can play a crucial role. To the extent that physicians faithfully discharge their responsibilities of economic advocacy, patients will be learning, through each encounter with the medical system, about the costs of health care and about the ways in which their own chosen insurance plans meet, or fail to meet, their own needs. Beyond this, people can at least partly overcome the information challenge through group action. Consumers can collectively hire agents or sponsors to do much of their investigating, as for example to ensure that the health plans competing for their business provide quality care through efficient practices.[60]

Once a person has freely and knowledgeably made such choices, however, it is essential that he be held accountable for his own decisions. This means that, if the patient has opted against some particular form of care that he later needs or wants, he either must pay for that care himself or go without. If his plan explicitly refuses to cover experimental care[61] then he is not wronged if, when later his unexpected major illness can only be treated by an experimental drug, his insurer refuses to pay for it. The reality may seem harsh, yet it is the only way in which to make, and adhere to, an economically and medically rational health care system. Eddy notes the awkwardness:

> What? Not cover an intervention that has benefit, just because of its cost? That's heresy! No, it's not heresy; it is the connection of value and cost . . . a conscious comparison of whether some real value offered by an intervention is worth its costs, and a determination to live with the decision.[62]

Physicians

As noted at the beginning of this chapter, medicine's economic revolution is forcing us to reexamine all of medical ethics, not just economic arrangements. In light of all we have discussed, it would seem that physicians' obligations, just like patients', need to be recast. Much of that work has been done throughout this volume, but here we may highlight a few important points.

In some respects, physicians' duties must be conceived much more modestly than in the past. We have seen, for example, that physicians are not obligated to commandeer others' resources, to sacrifice their own interests without limit, or to take upon themselves all their patients' difficult decisions with all the attendant guilt.

In other respects, however, physicians' responsibilities must grow in the new and extraordinarily complex world of health care. Physicians now bear some duties that have not previously loomed large, such as economic advocacy, economic disclosure, and a close scrutiny of the institutions and economic structures with which they affiliate.

Furthermore, the autonomy and responsibility now ascribed to the patient do not erase his vulnerability. He still needs a powerful, knowledgeable friend[63] who can help him to understand his choices and the impact they may have on his life, and who can help him to secure the care to which he is entitled. The physician therefore remains a fiduciary with powerful, even if not limitless, duties to do his best for his patient.

Probably more than anything else, the revised ethic of medicine must emphasize communication. The patient cannot truly make his own decisions, nor rightly be held accountable for them, if he does not understand the options from which he is choosing. And generally his most important source of information will be his physician. This does not entail that physicians must delve ever more deeply into the biological minutiae of illnesses and of medical interventions. Such technicalities rarely enhance the patient's real appreciation of the decisions that confront him.

Rather, the physician needs to be more richly aware of the basic values that are at stake where decisions must be made. A choice between surgery and radiation for cancer of the larynx, for example, is not a choice between computations of rads and lengths of incisions. Rather, one must pit fundamental values about the quality of life against some very basic risk preferences: with laryngectomy one enjoys a bit higher chance for survival, but at the cost of forfeiting normal speech for the rest of one's life.[64]

Similarly, many of the most common medical maladies do not require urgent decisions about life and death, nor do they have a single correct answer. Rather, they carry a variety of treatment options, each with differing implications for quality of life. Wennberg and his colleagues, for example, have discovered that "[m]en differ in their degree of concern about the symptoms of benign prostatic hypertrophy. Even some severely symptomatic patients are not bothered very much by their condition and prefer watchful waiting to surgery."[65] Studies of these patients and others now tend to confirm the hypothesis that, "particularly when risks must be taken to reduce symptoms or improve the quality of life, patients tend to be more risk averse than physicians. Given an option, patients will on average select less invasive strategies than physicians."[66] In such situations, a "rational choice depends on the patient's active involvement in the decision, because the patient's attitudes and values are the key to making the right decision."[67]

These conversations must now expand to encompass economics. Economics does not mean "mere money" in some crass sense. Earned money represents a value that has been placed on one's labors, and spent money reflects the goals one pursues. Every decision requires value choices, because decisions about what one should do are never simply dictated by facts. One must evaluate those facts in light of goals and values. In medicine's economics, we must weigh some health goals against other health goals, and these against all the other things that we could do with our limited resources. Is the slightly greater potency of this antibiotic *worth* its substantially higher cost? Are its projected medical benefits *worth* the remote possibility of an anaphylactic reaction?

If the physician is to help patients through such choices he needs to engage not in perfunctory recitations of fact or lengthy iterations of listed options, but in careful conversation—conversation that will require the patient to contribute actively and not stand passively by.[68] Because patients do remain vulnerable and in many cases very intimidated by the medical environment, the physician is also obligated to make such discussions as easy and inviting as possible. A perfunctory "Got any questions?" asked with one hand on the door knob and one foot out the door will not suffice. The physician must strive to elicit the patient's real concerns—the ones he may be too embarrassed to raise or too confused yet to have identified—in order to engage him in the kind of vigorous dialogue that is essential if all the important benefits and burdens of care are to be realized.[69]

CONCLUSION

Medicine's economic revolution can be a tremendous force for positive change. As we must now reckon with the enormous complexity of health care financing and delivery, and bid farewell to the insular, dyadic relationship between physician and patient, we can begin explicitly to put health care back into its broader context, the community as a whole. We can reject the atomism that tried to separate a person's health care choices from their economic and social implications for family, for society. It was born of a strange conception that saw human autonomy solely as unfettered freedom. To reinsert responsibility and insist that patients be regarded as autonomous in the full, real, responsible sense of the term reinvokes the broader perspective we need, for moral valuation and moral obligation can only be understood as social phenomena.

Medicine's economic revolution also provides enormous opportunity. In the past, when virtually unlimited payment for health care allowed us to escape making priority choices, we were able, even if only for a while, to avoid thinking about some important values. The economic challenges we now face will force us to ask, openly and carefully, just what we prize, not only in our health care, but in the other goals we may embrace as individuals and as a society. We have the opportunity to create a new order, one more consciously chosen, and chosen not just by a few to impose on the rest, but created by all who produce, pay for, or receive health care. It is an opportunity not to be missed.

NOTES

1. See, e.g., *Salgo v. Stanford*, 1957; *Natanson v. Kline*, 1960; *Cobbs v. Grant*, 1972; *Canterbury v. Spence*, 1972.
2. Kass, 1990; Veatch, 1981; Beauchamp and Childress, 1989.
3. Beauchamp and Childress, 1989, p. 68; see also Veatch, 1981; President's Commission, 1982, p. 44 ff.
4. Beauchamp and Childress, 1989, p. 71–72; Childress, 1990; Katz, 1984; Veatch, 1981; Morreim, 1983(b).
5. Katz, 1984; Kass, 1990; Childress, 1990.
6. Churchill, 1987, p. 20 ff.; Smith and Newton, 1984, p. 46.
7. Angell, 1985; Veatch, 1986.
8. This issue is discussed in Brett and McCullough, 1986.
9. Bovbjerg, Held, and Diamond, 1987; Butler and Haislmaier, 1989, p. 28.
10. Hotchkiss, 1987, p. 947.
11. Daniels, 1987, p. 71.

12. *Meinhard v. Salmon*, 1928.
13. Morreim, 1989(c); Morreim, 1987.
14. Hardwig, 1990.
15. For further discussion see Strong, 1984.
16. Ackerman, 1989.
17. Hardwig, 1990, pp. 6–7; Smith and Newton, 1984, p. 56.
18. Areen, 1988; Moore, 1989.
19. Engelhardt, 1986; President's Commission, 1982, p. 46. Note, although the President's Commission does mention responsibility as playing an important role in autonomy ("individuals define their own values . . . are capable of creating their own character and of taking responsibility for the kind of person they are"), this reference stands alone amid the more familiar focus upon autonomy-as-freedom.
20. Only rather recently do we find commentators more explicitly discussing patients' responsibilities as part of an analysis of their autonomy. See, e.g., Hardwig, 1990; Menzel, 1990.
21. Ingelfinger, 1980, pp. 1509–10; Paris, Crone, and Reardon, 1990, p. 1013.
22. Engelhardt, 1986, p. 275.
23. Sprung and Winnick, 1989, at 1352 (italics added).
24. Wolf, 1990, p. 209. Note, it is also common for physicians to make decisions on the patient's behalf on the grounds that this is (allegedly) what the patient wants; see Katz, 1984, p. 125.
25. Ingelfinger, 1980, p. 1509–10.
26. For a useful discussion of this concept see Erde, 1989.
27. For a discussion and critique of nondirective genetic counseling, see Yarborough, Scott, and Dixon, 1989.
28. Physicians also have been assigned rather extraordinary levels of responsibility in law. Law has long viewed the physician, in many circumstances at least, as being like the captain of the ship. That is, he is seen to be responsible not only for his own actions, but as well for actions of allied health care workers assisting him. In part, this concept arose because physicians do have legitimate duties to supervise those who work under them. But in part, the doctrine has simply provided a "handle" whereby patients could more easily recover damages for injuries in cases where other channels for recovery were unlikely to succeed. The doctrine of charitable immunity, for example, meant that indigent patients could not sue a charitable hospital even for injuries due to negligence. Where this applied, the "captain of the ship" doctrine enabled the patient to recover damages by suing the physician instead. While the "captain of the ship" doctrine has lost much of its earlier force in recent years, physicians continue to bear legal responsibility for actions and events considerably beyond their own professional conduct. The "borrowed servant" doctrine is now more likely to be invoked than the "cap-

tain" doctrine. See Areen, 1988, p. 44. We have also seen another substantial imposition of legal responsibility, above, as physicians may bear legal liability for below-standard use of medical and monetary resources, even though they do not always own or control the use of those resources.

29. Butler and Haislmaier, 1989, p. 28.

30. Katz, 1984, pp. 87, 125.

31. Engelhardt, 1986, p. 184–92 ff.

32. Though we cannot delve too deeply here into the economic changes in mental health care, it is interesting to note that, so long as there is fairly hefty reimbursement for mental health care, it may be profitable for certain providers to declare as many forms of conduct as possible to be diseases, so that they can be treated and reimbursed. These economic pressures to expand the concept of mental illness and disorder have ominous implications for human autonomy. See Morreim, 1990(a); see also Ritchie, 1989; Weithorn, 1988.

33. Callahan, 1982, p. 51.

34. Churchill, 1987, p. 20 ff.; Hardwig, 1990, p. 7.

35. Cook-Deegan, 1988, p. 127.

36. Moore, 1989.

37. We will consider persons with impaired capacity below.

38. See Feinberg, 1973, p. 59, for a discussion of *in rem* versus *in personam* rights and (by extension) duties.

39. To presume that wherever a decision is difficult, or its consequences unfortunate, others must make the decision and bear its consequences is rather like the "deep pocket" approach we find in tort law, wherein we seem to presume that if someone is injured and it is not his own fault, someone else who is better able to absorb the costs must pay—even if that other party bears very little fault.

40. Morreim, 1983(b).

41. Komaroff, 1990.

42. See also Hardwig, 1990, p. 8.

43. Miller, 1983.

44. Such decision responsibilities may also include lifestyle choices. These become increasingly important as more is known about the effects of voluntary behaviors such as smoking and nutrition habits upon one's overall health. While one's genetic endowment and many environmental factors are clearly beyond one's control, still there is much that lies within the province of personal choice and responsibility. See Spicker, 1988, p. 169; Churchill, 1987, p. 25; Katz, 1984, p. 154; Menzel, 1990. One can be more careful about a variety of known health risks by avoiding such obvious hazards as smoking and excessive drinking, following a better diet, and exercising regularly. Actually holding persons responsible for the effects of their lifestyle choices is admittedly difficult, as there are formidable obstacles to determining the

causal etiology of any given choice-related health problem. One's lung cancer, for example, may be clearly related to his long habit of heavy cigarette smoking, yet that same person may also have a genetic predisposition to develop cancer, or may have worked in a coal mine, thus making it difficult to determine just exactly what causal role his smoking played. In cases of substance abuse we may not even be able to agree whether the substance habit was the product of the person's free choice, or whether it is fully the product of forces outside the person's control.

Further, even if we agree that some illnesses are at least partly voluntarily self-induced, it can be a challenge to forge an appropriate social response. We may feel deeply reluctant to punish someone who is seriously ill by denying care on the grounds that his illness is his own fault. And we may be unable to detect the illicit behavior without extraordinarily intrusive means, such as spying on people in their homes or invading their bodies to do serological studies or gather other evidence of "wrongdoing."

Still, the admitted difficulties of ascribing causality and fixing social remedies do not preclude us from acknowledging that persons can and do exercise considerable control over their own health and welfare and that competent persons ought to select lifestyles that do not cause undue burdens to others.

45. Butler and Haislmaier, 1989, p. 42 ff.

46. Eddy, 1990(b).

47. For an excellent exposition of this line of reasoning, see Menzel, 1990, p. 10 ff., 32 ff. Although I quite agree with Menzel's arguments that we are respecting autonomy when we hold a person to the consequences of his own prior consent, I am not entirely willing to embrace his further view that, where we cannot secure the actual prior consent of an individual, the presumed consent of groups of people permit us to infer what a particular individual would have chosen. Menzel can probably move safely from a person's clear, actual prior consent to a presumed consent based on the known values and goals of that person. Such inferences are made, for example, when a patient has become incapacitated and his family must decide, based on their knowledge of him, whether he would or would not want aggressive medical care (see Menzel, p. 31). However, it is a large step from there to a broad claim about what some particular group of people would want, as for example where we assume in an ascription of metaconsent that rational poor persons might prudently wish to forgo access to the most exotic medical care in favor of retaining more money for the expenses of daily living. And it is a still larger step to infer from such a broad generalization to the presumed preferences of any given member of that group, if thereby we say that "rational poor persons would prefer this sort of health plan, so we will apply it to Jones." At this point, we have essentially removed ourselves completely from any real reliance on actual consent, in favor of some view about what someone in that situation surely ought to choose. Because actual choices are morally indispensable to the notion of rationing based on persons' autonomous, responsible decisions, it is essential that our national health policy strive to enhance patients' active involvement in shaping various health plan options and selecting among them.

48. Fleck, 1990, pp. 113–14.

49. Butler and Haislmaier, 1989, pp. 26–27.

50. Currently, many patients have very little choice among or influence over their health care plans. While the corporate employee may have a few choices among basic programs, often there is no opportunity to negotiate the contents of those programs or to shape the ways in which cost-care trade-offs are made. Insurance plans, for example, are largely contracts of adhesion in which the potential subscriber must simply take or leave what is offered. In some cases this lack of a rich spectrum of choices is a function of insurers' marketing practices (many benefit plans are designed to satisfy providers more than patients), but in other cases limits are a function of existing insurance law. Some states' laws mandating that certain benefits be covered in all health insurance, for example, prevent insurers from offering more flexible insurance options. See Butler and Haislmaier, 1989, pp. 6–15, 23, 28–31.

51. See, e.g., Enthoven and Kronick, 1989(a); Enthoven and Kronick, 1989(b); Himmelstein et al., 1989; Relman, 1989(a), pp. 117–18; Iglehart, 1990; Levey and Hill, 1989; Todd, 1989; Welch, 1989.

52. Enthoven and Kronick, 1989(a); Enthoven and Kronick, 1989(b); Enthoven, 1978(a); Enthoven, 1978(b).

53. Butler and Haislmaier, 1989; Menzel, 1990; Havighurst, 1986(c), p. 713 ff.

54. Fleck, 1990, p. 115 ff.; Relman, 1990.

55. Just how one would specify which services are the required minimum, and which should be regarded as optional is, of course, a challenging question that lies beyond the scope of this volume. It is a problem for anyone who recommends universal access to health care, whether or not one favors a consumer choice approach, since one must eventually specify to what everyone ought to have access.

56. For further discussion of contractual alternatives to tort, see Morreim, 1987; Morreim, 1989(c), and references cited there.

57. Butler and Haislmaier, 1989.

58. See Grumet, 1989; Abraham, 1981; see also Morreim, 1990(c) and Stern, 1983, for a discussion of "bad faith breach of contract," a legal doctrine that originated in insurance law, to address cases in which insurers deliberately attempt to sidestep their obligations.

59. Stern, 1983.

60. See, e.g., Havighurst, 1986(c), p. 714, 722; Enthoven, 1978(a); Enthoven, 1978(b); Enthoven and Kronick, 1989(a); Enthoven and Kronick, 1989(b).

61. We must also assume that the plan provides quite a clear definition of what sorts of care are to count as experimental. This problem has adversely affected some patients who expect to receive, e.g., the latest treatment for cancer, only to be told by their insurers that it is experimental and therefore not covered.

62. Eddy, 1990(b), p. 1739.

63. Fried, 1983.

64. McNeil, Weichselbaum, and Pauker, 1981.

65. Wennberg, 1990, p. 1202.

66. Ibid., p. 1203.

67. Ibid., p. 1202.

68. Katz, 1984.

69. For rich and practical discussions of how physicians can go about improving their communication with patients, see Katz, 1984; Cassell, 1985(a); Cassell, 1985(b).

References

BOOKS AND ARTICLES

Aaron, H. J., and W. B. Schwartz. 1984. *The painful prescription: Rationing hospital care*. Washington, D.C. Brookings Institution.

———. 1985. Hospital cost control: A bitter pill to swallow. *Harvard Business Review* 64:160–67.

Abraham, K. S. 1981. Judge-made law and judge-made insurance: Honoring the reasonable expectations of the insured. *Virginia Law Review* 67:1151–99.

Abraham, L. 1989. Specialties race against payers to set standards. *American Medical News* January 6:17, 19.

Abrams, F. R. 1986. Patient advocate or secret agent? *Journal of the American Medical Association* 256:1784–85.

Ackerman, T. F. 1989. An ethical framework for the practice of paying research subjects. *IRB: A Review of Human Subjects Research* 11(4):1–4.

Alderman, R. M. 1989. The business or medicine—Health care providers, physicians, and the deceptive trade practices act. *Houston Law Review* 26:109–43.

Altman, S. H., and M. A. Rodwin. 1988. Halfway competitive markets and ineffective regulation: The American health care system. *Journal of Health Politics, Policy and Law* 13(2):323–39.

American College of Physicians. 1990. Therapeutic substitution and formulary systems. *Annals of Internal Medicine* 113:160–63.

American Medical Association. 1986. *Current opinions of the council on ethical and judicial affairs*. Chicago: American Medical Association.

American Society of Internal Medicine. 1987. *Contracting guidelines for internists*. Washington, D.C.: American Society of Internal Medicine.

Andrulis, D. P., V. S. Beers, J. D. Bentley, and L. S. Gage. 1987. The provision of financing of medical care for AIDS patients in US public and private teaching hospitals. *Journal of the American Medical Association* 258:1343–46.

Andrulis, D. P., V. B. Weslowski, and L. S. Gage. 1989. The 1987 US hospital AIDS survey. *Journal of the American Medical Association* 262:784–94.

Angell, M. 1985. Cost containment and the physician. *Journal of the American Medical Association* 254:1203–07.

Areen, J. 1988. Legal intrusions on physician independence. In *The physician as captain of the ship: A critical reappraisal*, ed. N. M. P. King, L. R. Churchill, and A. W. Cross, pp. 39–66, Dordrecht: Reidel.

Aristotle. 1985. *Aristotle*. trans. Terence Irwin. Nicomachaen Ethics. Indianapolis: Hackett.

Arno, P. S. 1987. The economic impact of AIDS. *Journal of the American Medical Association* 258:1376–77.

Arras, J. D. 1988. The fragile web of responsibility: AIDS and the duty to treat. *Hastings Center Report* (Special Supplement) 18(2):10–20.

Astrachan, J. H., and B. M. Astrachan. 1989. Medical practice in organized settings. *Archives of Internal Medicine* 149:1509–13.

Avorn, J. L. 1986. Medicine, health, and the geriatric transformation. *Daedalus* 115:211–25.

Baily, M. A. 1984. "Rationing" and American health policy. *Journal of Health Politics, Policy and Law* 9:489–501.

Baily, M. 1986. Rationing medical care: Processes for defining adequacy. In *The Price of Health*, ed. G. Agich and C. Begley, pp. 165–84, Dordrecht: Reidel.

Banta, H. D., and S. B. Thacker. 1990. The case for reassessment of health care technology. *Journal of the American Medical Association* 264:235–40.

Beauchamp, T. L., and J. F. Childress. 1989. *Principles of biomedical ethics*, 3rd ed. New York: Oxford University Press.

Begley, C. 1986. Physicians and cost control. In *The Price of Health*, ed. G. Agich and C. Begley, pp. 227–44, Dordrecht: Reidel.

———. 1987. Prospective payment and medical ethics. *The Journal of Medicine and Philosophy* 12:107–122.

Benn, S. I. 1967. Justice. In *The Encyclopedia of Philosophy*, ed. P. Edwards., pp. 298–02, New York: Macmillan Publishing Co.

Berenson, R. A. 1987. In a doctor's wallet. *The New Republic* 196: 11–13.

———. 1989. A physician's reflections. *Hastings Center Report* 19(1):12–15.

Berki, S. E. 1985. DRGs, incentives, hospitals, and physicians. *Health Affairs* 4(4):70–76.

Berry, M. J. 1990. Analyze your practice's collection management system. *American Medical News* (October 12):20–21.

Black, H. C., J. R. Nolan, and M. J. Connolly. 1983. *Black's law dictionary*. St. Paul: West.

Blendon, R. J. 1986. The problems of cost, access, and distribution of medical care. *Daedalus* 115:119–35.

Blendon, R. J., L. H. Aiken, H. E. Freeman, et al. 1986. Uncompensated care by hospitals or public insurance for the poor. *The New England Journal of Medicine* 314:1160–63.

Blum, J. 1991. Economic credentialing: A new twist in hospital–physician appraisal processes. *Journal of Legal Medicine* 12:427–75.

Blumstein, J. F., and F. A. Sloan. 1981. Redefining Government's role in health care: Is a dose of competition just what the doctor should order? *Vanderbilt Law Review* 34:849–26.

Board of Trustees Report. 1986. A proposal for financing health care of the elderly. *Journal of the American Medical Association* 256:3379–82.

Board of Trustees Report. 1989. AMA policy on the resource-based relative value scale and related issues. *Journal of the American Medical Association* 261:2386–88.

Bock, R. S. 1988. The pressure to keep prices high at a walk-in clinic. *The New England Journal of Medicine* 319:785–87.

Bok, S. 1978, *Lying*. New York: Random House.

Borus, J. F. 1986. Coverage, care, cost, and outcome. *Journal of the American Medical Association* 256:1939.

Bovbjerg, R. R., P. J. Held, and L. H. Diamond. 1987. Provider–patient relations and treatment choice in the era of fiscal incentives: The case of the end-stage renal disease program. *The Milbank Quarterly* 65:177–203.

Bowen, O. R. 1987. Shattuck lecture—What is quality care? *The New England Journal of Medicine* 316:1578–80.

Boyle, J. F. 1984. Should we learn to say no? *Journal of the American Medical Association* 252:782–84.

Brailer, D. J., and D. B. Nash. 1986. Uncertainty and the future of young physicians. *Journal of the American Medical Association* 256:3391–92.

Brazil, P. 1986. Cost effective care is better care. *Hastings Center Report* 16(1): 7–8.

Brennan, T. A. 1987. Untangling causation issues in law and medicine: Hazardous substance litigation. *Annals of Internal Medicine* 107:741–47.

Brett, A. S. 1981. Hidden ethical issues in clinical decision analysis. *The New England Journal of Medicine* 305:1150–53.

Brett, A. S., and L. B. McCullough. 1986. When patients request specific interventions. *The New England Journal of Medicine* 315:1347–51.

Brock, D. W. 1986. Commentary: Implications of new physician payment methods for access to health care and physician fidelity to patients' interests. *Case Western Reserve Law Review* 36:760–77.

Brock, D. W., and A. E. Buchanan. 1987. The profit motive in medicine. *The Journal of Medicine and Philosophy* 12:1–35.

Brody, B. A. 1987. Justice and competitive markets. *The Journal of Medicine and Philosophy* 12:37–50.

Brody, H. 1987. Cost containment as professional challenge. *Theoretical Medicine* 8:5–17.

———. 1989. The physician–patient relationship. In *Medical Ethics*, ed. R. M. Veatch, pp. 65–91, Boston: Jones and Bartlett.

Brook, R. H. 1989. Practice guidelines and practicing medicine: Are they compatible? *Journal of the American Medical Association* 262:3027–30.

Brookes, B. 1989. The new health service in New Zealand. *Hastings Center Report* (Special Supplement) 19(4):13–15.

Buchanan, A. E. 1984. The right to a decent minimum of health care. *Philosophy and Public Affairs* 13:55–78.

———. 1985, Ethics, efficiency, and the market. Totowa: Rowman and Allenheld.

Burnum, J. F. 1987. Medical practice a la mode. *The New England Journal of Medicine* 317:1220–22.

Butler, C. 1985. Preferred provider organization liability for physician malpractice. *American Journal of Law and Medicine* 11:345–68.

Butler, S. M., and E. F. Haislmaier, eds. 1989. *Critical issues: A national health system for America*. Washington, D.C.: Heritage Foundation.

Callahan, D. 1982. The WHO definition of "health." In *Contemporary Issues in Bioethics*, ed. L. Walters, pp. 49–54, Belmont: Wadsworth.

———. 1986. Adequate health care and an aging society: Are they morally compatible? *Daedalus* 115:247–67.

———. 1990. Rationing medical progress: The way to affordable health care. *The New England Journal of Medicine* 322:1810–13.

Caplan, A. L. 1982. Mechanics on duty: The limits of a technical definition of moral expertise for work in applied ethics. *Canadian Journal of Philosophy*, Supplementary Volume 8:1–18.

———. 1983. Can applied ethics be effective in health care and should it strive to be? *Ethics* 93:311–19.

Capron, A. M. 1986. Containing health care costs: Ethical and legal implications of changes in the methods of paying physicians. *Case Western Reserve Law Review* 36:708–59.

Capron, A. M., and B. H. Gray. 1984. Between you and your doctor. *Wall Street Journal*, February 6.

Cassel, C. K. 1985. Doctors and allocation decisions: A new role in the new medicare. *Journal of Health Politics, Policy and Law* 10:549–64.

Cassell, E. J. 1981. Do justice, love mercy: The inappropriateness of the concept of justice applied to bedside decisions. In *Justice and Health Care*, ed. E. Shelp, pp. 75–82, Dordrecht: Reidel.

———. 1985(a), *Talking with patients* (Volume 1: The theory of doctor–patient communication). Cambridge: The MIT Press.

———. 1985(a), *Talking with patients* (Volume 2: Clinical techniques). Cambridge: The MIT Press.

———. 1986. The changing concept of the ideal physician. *Daedalus* 115:185–208.

Chalmers, T. C. 1988. PET scans and technology assessment. *Journal of the American Medical Association* 260:2713–15.

Chassin, M. R., R. H. Brook, R. E. Park et al. 1986. Variations in the use of medical and surgical services by the medicare population. *The New England Journal of Medicine* 314:285–90.

Childress, J. F. 1990. The place of autonomy in bioethics. *Hastings Center Report* 20(1):12–17.

Churchill, L. R. 1987. *Rationing health care in America: Perceptions and principles of justice*. Notre Dame: University of Notre Dame Press.

Cluff, L. E. 1986. America's romance with medicine and medical science. *Daedalus* 115:137–59.

Cohen, C. 1989. Militant morality: Civil disobedience and bioethics. *Hastings Center Report* 19(6):23–25.

Cook-Deegan, R. M. 1988. The physician and technological change. In *The Physician as Captain of the Ship: A Critical Reappraisal*, eds. N. M. P. King, L. R. Churchill and A. W. Cross, pp. 125–58, Dordrecht: Reidel.

Council on Long-range Planning and Development. 1986. Health care in transition. *Journal of the American Medical Association* 256:3384–90.

Council on Scientific Affairs. 1988. Positron emission tomography—A new approach to brain chemistry. *Journal of the American Medical Association* 260:2704–10.

Curran, W. J., and G. B. Moseley III. 1975. The malpractice experience of health maintenance organizations. *Northwestern University Law Review* 70:69–89.

D'Anastasio, M. 1987. Soviet health system, despite early claims is riddled by failures. *Wall Street Journal*, August 18:1,8.

Daniels, N. 1985. *Just health care.* Cambridge: Cambridge University Press.

———. 1986. Why saying no to patients in the United States is so hard. *The New England Journal of Medicine* 314:1380–83.

———. 1987. The ideal advocate and limited resources. *Theoretical Medicine* 8:69–80.

Dans, P. E., J. P. Weiner, and S. E. Otter. 1985. Peer review organizations: Promises and potential pitfalls. *The New England Journal of Medicine* 313:1131–37.

Davis, K. 1986. Aging and the health-care system: Economic and structural issues. *Daedalus* 115:227–46.

Dawson, J. H. 1987. Practice variations: A challenge for physicians. *Journal of the American Medical Association* 258:2570.

Demkovich, L. E. 1986. Controlling health care costs at General Motors. *Health Affairs* 5(3):58–67.

Detre, T. 1987. The future of psychiatry. *American Journal of Psychiatry* 144:621–25.

Dougherty, C. J. 1988, *American health care: Realities, rights, and reforms.* New York: Oxford University Press.

Duff, R. S. 1988. Unshared and shared decisionmaking: Reflections on helplessness and healing. In *The physician as captain of the ship: A critical reappraisal*, eds. N. M. P. King, L. R. Churchill and A. W. Cross, pp. 191–222, Dordrecht: Reidel.

Eddy, D. M. 1982. Clinical policies and the quality of clinical practice. *The New England Journal of Medicine* 307:343–47.

———. 1984. Variations in physician practice: The role of uncertainty. *Health Affairs* 3(2):74–89.

———. 1990(a). What do we do about costs? *Journal of the American Medical Association* 264:1161, 1165, 1169, 1170.

———. 1990. Connecting value and costs: Whom do we ask, and what do we ask them? *Journal of the American Medical Association* 264:1737–39.

Egdahl, R. H. 1983. Ways for surgeons to increase the efficiency of their use of hospitals. *The New England Journal of Medicine* 309:1184–87.

———. 1987. Maintain quality when cutting health costs. *Wall Street Journal*, 5 January 1987.

Egdahl, R. H., and C. H. Taft. 1986. Financial incentives to physicians. *The New England Journal of Medicine* 315:59–61.

Eisenberg, J. A. 1985. The internist as gatekeeper. *Annals of Internal Medicine* 102:537–43.

Elkowitz, A. 1987. Health care: Discrimination against the rich? *Bioethics* 1:272–74.

Ellwood Jr., P. M. 1983(a). Meshing hospitals and physicians provides mutual benefits. *Hospitals* 57:63–64.

———. 1983(b). When MDs meet DRGs. *Hospitals* 57:62.

———. 1988. Shattuck lecture—outcomes management: A technology of patient experience. *The New England Journal of Medicine* 318:1549–56.

Emanuel, E. 1988. Do physicians have an obligation to treat patients with AIDS? *The New England Journal of Medicine* 318:1686–90.

———. 1986. *The foundations of bioethics*, Oxford: Oxford University Press.

Engelhardt, H. T., and M. A. Rie. 1986. Intensive care units, scarce resources, and conflicting principles of justice. *Journal of the American Medical Association* 255:1159–64.

———. 1988. Morality for the medical industrial complex. *The New England Journal of Medicine* 319:1086–89.

Enthoven, A. C. 1978(a). Consumer-choice health plan: Inflation and inequity in health care today: Alternatives for cost control and an analysis of proposals for national health insurance, Part One. *The New England Journal of Medicine* 298:650–58.

———. 1978(b). Consumer-choice health plan: A national-health-insurance proposal based on regulated competition in the private sector. *The New England Journal of Medicine* 298:709–20.

———. 1989. Effective management of competition in the FEHBP. *Health Affairs* 8(3):33–50.

Enthoven, A., and R. Kronick. 1989(a). A consumer-choice health plan for the 1990s: Universal health insurance in a system designed to promote quality and economy, Part I. *The New England Journal of Medicine* 320:29–37.

———. 1989(b). A consumer-choice health plan for the 1990s: Universal health insurance in a system designed to promote quality and economy, Part II. *The New England Journal of Medicine* 320:94–101.

Epstein, A. M. 1990. The outcomes movement—Will it get us where we want to go? *The New England Journal of Medicine* 323:266–70.

Erde, E. L. 1989. Studies in the explanation of issues in biomedical ethics: (II) On "on play[ing] God", etc. *The Journal of Medicine and Philosophy* 14:593–616.

Evans, R. G. 1986. Finding the levers, finding the courage: Lessons from cost containment in North America. *Journal of Health Politics, Policy and Law* 11(4):585–615.

Evans, R. W. 1983(a). Health care technology and the inevitability of resource allocation and rationing decisions: Part I. *Journal of the American Medical Association* 249:2047–53.

———. 1983(b). Health care technology and the inevitability of resource allocation and rationing decisions: Part II. *Journal of the American Medical Association* 249:2208–19.

Feinberg, J. 1973, *Social Philosophy.* Englewood Cliffs: Prentice-Hall.

Feinglass, J. 1987. Variations in physician practice and covert rationing. *Theoretical Medicine* 8:31–45.

Feldman, S. R., and T. M. Ward. 1979. Psychotherapeutic injury: Reshaping the implied contract as an alternative to malpractice. *North Carolina Law Review* 58:65–97.

Fine M. W., and J. H. Sunshine. 1986. Malpractice reform through consumer choice and consumer education: Are new concepts marketable? *Law and Contemporary Problems* 49:213–22.

Fisek, N. H. 1989. In Turkey, new goals for health care. *Hastings Center Report* (Special Supplement) 19(4):15–17.

Fleck, L. M. 1987. DRGs: Justice and the invisible rationing of health care resources. *The Journal of Medicine and Philosophy* 12:165–196.

———. 1989(a). Just health care (I): Is beneficence enough? *Theoretical Medicine* 10:167–82.

———. 1989(b). Just health care (II): Is equality too much? *Theoretical Medicine* 10:301–10.

———. 1990. Justice, HMOs, and the invisible rationing of health care resources. *Bioethics* 4:97–120.

Freedman, S. A. 1985. Megacorporate health care. *The New England Journal of Medicine* 312:579–82.

Freedman, S. A., B. R. Klepper, R. P. Duncan, and S.P. Bell. 1988. Coverage of the uninsured and underinsured. *The New England Journal of Medicine* 318:843–47.

Freiman, M. P. 1984. Cost sharing lessons from the private sector. *Health Affairs* 3(4):85–93.

Fried, C. 1975. Rights and health care—Beyond equity and efficiency. *The New England Journal of Medicine* 293:241–45.

———. 1981. *Contract as promise.* Cambridge: Harvard University Press.

———. 1983. The lawyer as friend: The moral foundations of the lawyer–client relation. In *Moral Responsibility and the Professions*, eds. B. Baumrin and B. Freedman. New York: Haven Publications.

Friedman, E. 1987. Public hospitals often face unmet capital needs, underfunding, uncompensated patient-care costs. *Journal of the American Medical Association* 257:1698–1701.

Fuchs, V. R. 1984. The "rationing" of medical care. *New England Journal of Medicine* 311:1572–73.

———. 1986. *The health economy.* Cambridge: Harvard University Press.

———. 1987. The counterrevolution in health care financing. *The New England Journal of Medicine* 316:1154–56.

Furrow, B. R. 1986. Medical malpractice and cost containment: Tightening the screws. *Case Western Reserve Law Review* 36:985–1032.

———. 1988. The ethics of cost-containment: Bureaucratic medicine and the doctor as patient-advocate. *Notre Dame Journal of Law, Ethics and Public Policy* 3:187–225.

Gabbard, G. 1985. The role of compulsiveness in the normal physician. *Journal of the American Medical Association* 254:2926–29.

Gabel, J., C. Jajich-Toth, K. Williams et al. 1987. The commercial health insurance industry in transition. *Health Affairs* 6(3):46–60.

Gage, L. S. 1987. Our nation's great public hospitals. *Journal of the American Medical Association* 257:1942–43.

Geyelin, M. 1990. HMOs' malpractice immunity is fading, *Wall Street Journal* February 1, pp. B–1, B–7.

Gillick, M. R. 1987. The impact of health maintenance organizations on geriatric care. *Annals of Internal Medicine* 106:139–43.

Ginzberg, E. 1983. Cost containment—imaginary and real. *The New England Journal of Medicine* 308:1220–24.

———. 1986. The destabilization of health care. *The New England Journal of Medicine* 315:757–61.

———. 1987. A hard look at cost containment. *The New England Journal of Medicine* 316:1151–54.

———. 1990. High-tech medicine and rising health care costs. *Journal of the American Medical Association* 263:1820–22.

Gleick, J. 1987. *Chaos.* New York: Penguin Books.

Glenn, J. K., F. H. Lawler, and M. S. Hoerl. 1987. Physician referrals in a competitive environment. *Journal of the American Medical Association* 258:1920–23.

Goldman, A. 1984. Ethical issues in advertising. In *Just Business: New Introductory Essays in Business Ethics,* ed. T. Regan, pp. 235–71, New York: Random House.

Goldman, L., E. F. Cook, D. A. Brand et al. 1988. A computer protocol to predict myocardial infarction in emergency department patients with chest pain. *The New England Journal of Medicine* 318:797–803.

Goldsmith, J. C. 1986. The US health care system in the year 2000. *Journal of the American Medical Association* 256:3371–75.

Gorovitz, S., and A. MacIntyre. 1976. Toward a theory of medical fallibility. *The Journal of Medicine and Philosophy* 1:51–71.

Graham, G. 1987. The doctor, the rich, and the indigent. *The Journal of Medicine and Philosophy* 12:51–61.

Gray, B. H. 1983. An introduction to the new health care for profit. In *The New Health Care for Profit,* ed. B.H. Gray, pp. 1–16, Washington: National Academy Press.

Gray, B. H. and M. J. Field, eds. 1989. *Controlling costs and changing patient care?: The role of utilization management.* Washington: National Academy Press (Institute of Medicine).

Greenfield, S. 1989. The state of outcome research: Are we on target? *The New England Journal of Medicine* 320:1142–43.

Greenspan, A. M., H. R. Kay, B. C. Berger et al. 1988. Incidence of unwarranted implantation of permanent cardiac pacemakers in a large medical population. *The New England Journal of Medicine* 318:158–63.

Grumet, G. W. 1989. Health care rationing through inconvenience: The third party's secret weapon. *The New England Journal of Medicine* 321:607–11.

Gutheil, T. G., J. Bursztajn, and A. Brodsky. 1984. Malpractice prevention through the sharing of uncertainty. *The New England Journal of Medicine* 311:49–51.

Gutmann, A. 1983. For and against equal access to health care. In *Securing Access to Health Care*, Volume Two, ed. President's Commission for the Study of Ethical Problems in Medicine and Biomedical 'and Behavioral Research, pp. 51–66, Washington: U.S. Government Printing Office.

Hall, M. A. 1988. Institutional control of physician behavior: Legal barriers to health care cost containment. *University of Pennsylvania Law Review* 137:431–536.

———. 1989. The malpractice standard under health care cost containment. *Law, Medicine and Health Care* 17:347–55.

Hall, M. A., and I. M. Ellman. 1990. *Health Care Law and Ethics*. St. Paul: West.

Halper, T. 1987. DRGs and the idea of a just price. *The Journal of Medicine and Philosophy* 12:155–64.

Hardin, G. 1968. The tragedy of the commons. *Science* 162:1243–48.

Hardison, J. E. 1979. To be complete. *The New England Journal of Medicine* 300:193–94.

Hardwig, J. 1987. Robin Hoods and Good Samaritans: The role of patients in health care distribution. *Theoretical Medicine* 8:47–59.

———. 1990. What about the family? *Hastings Center Report* 20(2):5–10.

Havighurst, C. C. 1986(a). Professional peer review and the antitrust laws. *Case Western Reserve Law Review* 36:1117–69.

———. 1986(b). Altering the applicable standard of care. In *Law and Contemporary Problems*, pp. 265–76, Durham: Duke University School of Law.

———. 1986(c). The changing locus of decision making in the health care sector. *Journal of Health Politics, Policy and Law* 11:697–735.

Hemenway, D., A. Killen, S. Cashman et al. 1990. Physicians' responses to financial incentives: Evidence from a for-profit ambulatory center. *The New England Journal of Medicine* 322:1059–63.

Hernried, J., L. Binder, and P. Hernried. 1990. Effect of student loan indebtedness and repayment on resident physicians' cash flow: An analytic model. *Journal of the American Medical Association* 263:1102–05.

Hershey, N. 1986. Fourth-party audit organizations: Practical and legal considerations. *Law, Medicine and Health Care* 14:54–65.

Hiatt, H. H. 1975. Protecting the medical commons: Who is responsible? *The New England Journal of Medicine* 293:235–41.

———. 1987. *America's Health in the Balance*. New York: Harper & Row.

Hillman, A. L. 1987. Financial incentives for physicians in HMOs: Is there a conflict of interest? *The New England Journal of Medicine* 317:1743–48.

———. 1990. Health maintenance organizations, financial incentives, and physicians' judgments. *Annals of Internal Medicine* 112:891–93.

Hillman, A. L., M. V. Pauly, and J. J. Kerstein. 1989. How do financial incentives affect physicians' clinical decisions and the financial performance of health maintenance organizations? *The New England Journal of Medicine* 321:86–92.

Hillman, B. J., C. A. Joseph, M. R. Mabry et al. 1990. Frequency and costs of diagnostic imaging in office practice—A comparison of self-referring and radiologist-referring physicians. *The New England Journal of Medicine* 323:1604–08.

Himmelstein, D. U., S. Woolhandler et al. 1989. A national health program for the United States: A physicians' proposal. *The New England Journal of Medicine* 320:102–08.

Hirshorn, M. W. 1986. Some doctors assail quality of treatment provided by HMOs. *Wall Street Journal*, September 16, pp. 1, 21.

Holder, A. R. 1978. *Medical malpractice law* (2nd edition). New York: John Wiley.

Hotchkiss, W. S. 1987. Doctor as patient advocate. *Journal of the American Medical Association* 258:947–48.

Hsiao, W. C., P. Braun, E. R. Becker, and S. R. Thomas. 1987. The resource-based relative value scale. *Journal of the American Medical Association* 258:799–802.

Hsiao, W. C., P. Braun, D. Dunn et al. 1988. Results and policy implications of the resource-based relative-value study. *The New England Journal of Medicine* 319:881–88.

Hsiao, W. C., P. Braun, D. Yntema et al. 1988. Estimating physicians' work for a resource-based relative-value scale. *The New England Journal of Medicine* 319:835–41.

Hull, J. B. 1984. Hospitals and doctors clash over efforts by administrators to cut medicare costs. *Wall Street Journal*, January 19.

Hume, D. 1888, *A treatise of human nature* (1973 printing), ed. L. A. Selby-Bigge. Oxford: Oxford University Press.

Hyman, D. A., and J. V. Williamson. 1988. Fraud and abuse: Regulatory alternatives in a "competitive" health care era. *Loyola University Law Journal* 19:1133–97.

Iezzoni, L. I., and M. A. Moskowitz. 1986. Clinical overlap among medical diagnosis-related groups. *Journal of the American Medical Association* 255:927–29.

Iglehart, J. K. 1983. Medicaid turns to prepaid managed care. *The New England Journal of Medicine* 308:976–80.

———. 1985(a). Medicare turns to HMOs, *The New England Journal of Medicine* 312:132–36.

———. 1985(b). The Administration's assault on domestic spending and the threat to health care programs. *The New England Journal of Medicine* 312:525–28.

———. 1987(a). The political contest over health care resumes. *The New England Journal of Medicine* 316:639–44.

———. 1987(b). Second thoughts about HMOs for medicare patients. *The New England Journal of Medicine* 316:1487–92.

———. 1987(c). Financing the struggle against AIDS. *The New England Journal of Medicine* 317:180–84.

———. 1990. The new law on medicare's payments to physicians. *The New England Journal of Medicine* 322:1247–52.

Ingelfinger, F. J. 1980. Arrogance. *The New England Journal of Medicine* 303:1507–11.

Institute of Medicine. 1986. Committee Report. In *For-profit enterprise in health care*, ed. B. H. Gray, pp. 127–204, Washington: National Academy Press.

Jackson, D. L., and S. Youngner. 1979. Patient autonomy and "death with dignity": Some clinical caveats. *The New England Journal of Medicine* 301:404–08.

Jacobson, P. D., and C.J. Rosenquist. 1988. The introduction of low-osmolar contrast agents in radiology. *Journal of the American Medical Association* 260:1586–92.

James, F. E. 1987(a). Blue Cross plans coverage limits on many tests. *Wall Street Journal*, April 1, p. 29.

———. 1987(b). Study lays groundwork for tying health costs to workers' behavior. *Wall Street Journal*, April 14, p. 35.

Jecker, N. S. 1990. Integrating medical ethics with normative theory: Patient advocacy and social responsibility. *Theoretical Medicine* 11:125–39.

Jennings, B., D. Callahan, and A.L. Caplan. 1988. Ethical challenges of chronic illness. *Hastings Center Report* 18(1) (Supp.):1–16.

Johns, R. J., and N. J. Fortuin. 1988. Clinical information and clinical problem solving. In *The Principles and Practice of Medicine*, 22nd (ed.), eds. A. M. Harvey, R. J. Johns, V. A. McKusick, A. H. Owens, and R. S. Ross, pp. 1–4, Norwalk: Appleton and Lange.

Jonsen, A. R. 1983. Watching the doctor. *The New England Journal of Medicine* 308:1531–35.

———. 1986. Bentham in a box: Technology assessment and health care allocation. *Law, Medicine and Health Care* 14:172–74.

Jonsen, A. R., and S. Toulmin. 1988, *The Abuse of Casuistry*. Berkeley: University of California Press.

Kant, I. 1785. *Foundation of the metaphysics of morals*, trans. L. W. Beck (ed.) (1959 edition). Indianapolis: Bobbs-Merrill.

Kapp, M. B. 1984. Legal and ethical implications of health care reimbursement by diagnosis related groups. *Law, Medicine and Health Care* 12:245–53.

Kass, L. R. 1990. Practicing ethics: Where's the action? *Hastings Center Report* 20(1):5–12.

Kassirer, J. P. 1989. Our stubborn quest for diagnostic certainty: A cause of excessive testing. *The New England Journal of Medicine* 320:1489–91.

Katz, J. 1984. *The silent world of doctor and patient*. New York: Free Press.

Kellermann, A. L., and T. F. Ackerman. 1988. Interhospital patient transfer: The case for informed consent. *The New England Journal of Medicine* 319:643–47.

Kellermann, A. L., and B. B. Hackman. 1988. Emergency department patient 'dumping': An analysis of interhospital transfers to the regional medical center at Memphis, Tennessee. *American Journal of Public Health* 78:1287–92.

Kemper, K. J. 1988. Medically inappropriate hospital use in a pediatric population. *The New England Journal of Medicine* 318:1033–37.

Kent, D. L., and E. B. Larson. 1988. Diagnostic technology assessments: Problems and prospects. *Annals of Internal Medicine* 108:759–61.

King, J. H., Jr. 1986. *The law of medical malpractice in a nutshell*, 2nd. ed. St. Paul: West.

Kinney, E. D., and M. M. Wilder. 1989. Medical standard setting in the current malpractice environment: Problems and possibilities. *University of California, Davis Law Review* 22:421–50.

Klein, R. 1989. From global rationing to target setting in the U.K. *Hastings Center Report* (Special Supplement) 19(4):3–7.

Knotterus, W. 1984. California Negotiated health care: Implications for malpractice liability. *San Diego Law Review* 21:455–76.

Komaroff, A. L. 1990. "Minor" illness symptoms: The magnitude of their burden and of our ignorance. *Archives of Internal Medicine* 150:1586–87.

Kosecoff, J., D. E. Kanouse, W. H. Rogers et al. 1987. Effects of the National Institutes of Health consensus development program on physician practice. *Journal of the American Medical Association* 258:2708–13.

Kusserow, R.P. 1989, *Financial Arrangements Between Physicians and Health Care Businesses*. Washington: U.S. Government Printing Office.

Lachs, M. S., J. L. Sindelar, and R. I. Horwitz. 1990. The forgiveness of coinsurance: Charity or cheating? *The New England Journal of Medicine* 322:1599–1602.

Larkin, H. 1990. Utilization review, special services earn some physicians a stipend. *American Medical News*, May 25, pp. 17, 20, 21.

Leaf, A. 1984. The doctor's dilemma—And society's too. *The New England Journal of Medicine* 310:718–20.

Lee, P. R., P. B. Ginsburg, L. B. LeRoy, and G. T. Hammons. 1989. The physician payment review commission report to Congress. *Journal of the American Medical Association* 261:2382–85.

Levey, S., and J. Hill. 1989. National health insurance—The triumph of equivocation. *New England Journal of Medicine* 321:1750–54.

Levinsky, N. G. 1984. The doctor's master. *The New England Journal of Medicine* 311:1573–75.

Levinson, D. F. 1987. Toward full disclosure of referral restrictions and financial incentives by prepaid health plans. *The New England Journal of Medicine* 317:1729–31.

Light, D. W. 1983. Is competition bad? *The New England Journal of Medicine* 309:1315–19.

Lister, J. 1986. Shattuck lecture—The politics of medicine in Britain and the United States. *The New England Journal of Medicine* 315:168–74.

———. 1989. Proposals for reform of the British national health service. *The New England Journal of Medicine* 320:877–80.

Lubell, A. 1987. Liquid gold creates safety, cost dilemma. *American Medical News*, October 9, pp. 26, 27, 28, 29, 30.

Luft, H. S. 1983. Economic incentives and clinical decisions. In *The New Health Care for Profit*, ed. B. H. Gray, pp. 103–23, Washington: National Academy Press.

Lundberg, G. A. 1983. Perseveration of laboratory test ordering: A syndrome affecting clinicians. *Journal of the American Medical Association* 249:639.

MacIntyre, A. 1981, *After virtue*. Notre Dame: University of Notre Dame Press.

MacNabb, D. G. C. 1967. Hume. In *The Encyclopedia of Philosophy*, ed. P. Edwards, pp. 74–90, New York: Macmillan.

Maloney, Jr., J. V., and K. Reemtsma. 1985. Cost containment by a naval armada. *The New England Journal of Medicine* 312:1713–14.

Marcus, S. A. 1984. Trade unionism for doctors: An idea whose time has come. *The New England Journal of Medicine* 311:1508–11.

Marmor, T. R. 1986. Commentary. *Case Western Reserve Law Review* 36:686–92.

Matsui, R. T. 1985. Medicare payment policy needs corrections. *Journal of the American Medical Association* 254:2454–55.

May, W. E. 1986. On ethics and advocacy. *Journal of the American Medical Association* 256:1786–87.

May, W. F. 1975. Code, covenant, contract, or philanthropy? *Hastings Center Report* 5(6):29–38.

McCarthy, C. M. 1988. Financing indigent care: Short- and long-term strategies. *Journal of the American Medical Association* 259:75.

McDowell, T. N. Jr. 1989. Physician self referral arrangements: Legitimate business or unethical "entrepreneurialism". *American Journal of Law and Medicine* 15(1):61–109.

McNeil, B. J., R. Weichselbaum, and S.G. Pauker. 1981. Speech and survival: Tradeoffs between quality and quantity of life in laryngeal cancer. *New England Journal of Medicine* 305:982–987.

Mechanic, D. 1986, *From advocacy to allocation: The evolving American health care system*. New York: Free Press.

Melnick, S. D., and L. L. Lyter. 1987. The negative impacts of increased concurrent review of psychiatric inpatient care. *Hospital and Community Psychiatry* 38(3):300–03.

Menzel, P. T. 1987. Economic competition in health care: A moral assessment. *The Journal of Medicine and Philosophy* 12:63–84.

———. 1990, *Strong medicine: The ethical rationing of health care*. New York: Oxford University Press.

Merken, G. 1989. Decoding hospital bills can make you sick. *Wall Street Journal*, May 10, A–22.

Meyer, H. 1987(a). Ob-Gyns quit Md. HMO to protest test payment plan. *American Medical News*, March 13, p. 15.

———. 1987(b). Suit blames HMO capitation for damaging quality of care. *American Medical News*, September 4, pp. 2, 46, 47.

———. 1987(c). Medical societies claim win in fight over HMO drug lists. *American Medical News*, December 18, pp. 2, 32.

———. 1988. 2 HMOs offer MD bonuses for high quality marks. *American Medical News*, March 11, pp. 4, 5.

———. 1989(a). Suit: HMO failed to disclose MD cost incentives. *American Medical News*, January 20, pp. 4, 5.

———. 1989(b). APA issues practice guidelines despite rift in its ranks. *American Medical News*, May 12, p. 10.

———. 1990. Cost sharing raises patient ire; does it reduce use? *American Medical News*, May 18, pp. 1, 42, 43.

Miller, F. H. 1983. Secondary income from recommended treatment: Should fiduciary principles constrain physician behavior? In *The new health care for profit*, ed. B. H. Gray, pp. 153–69, Washington: National Academy Press.

Mills, J. S. 1881, *Utilitarianism*, trans. ed. Oskar Piest, (1957 edition). Indianapolis: Bobbs-Merrill.

Mindell, B. 1988. IPCs establish beachhead in Cleveland. *American Medical News*, February 12, pp. 13, 18.

Mitchell, S. A., and J. R. Virts. 1986. Health Care cost containment: What is too much? *Health Affairs* 5(4):112–19.

Mold, J. W., and H. F. Stein. 1986. The cascade effect in the clinical care of patients. *The New England Journal of Medicine* 314:512–14.

Moore, C. 1989. Need for a patient advocate. *Journal of the American Medical Association* 262:259–60.

Moore, S. 1979. Cost containment through risk-sharing by primary-care physicians. *The New England Journal of Medicine* 300:1359–62.

Morreim, E. H. 1983(a). The philosopher in the clinical setting. *The Pharos* 46(1):2–6.

———. 1983(b). Three concepts of patient competence. *Theoretical Medicine* 4:231–51.

———. 1985(a). Cost containment: Issues of moral conflict and justice for physicians. *Theoretical Medicine* 6:257–79.

———. 1985(b). The MD and the DRG. *Hastings Center Report* 15(3):30–38.

———. 1986(a). Philosophy lessons from the clinical setting: Seven sayings that used to annoy me. *Theoretical Medicine* 7:47–63.

———. 1986(b). Commentary: Stratified scarcity and unfair liability. *Case Western Reserve Law Review* 36:1033–57.

———. 1987. Cost containment and the standard of medical care. *California Law Review* 75:1719–63.

———. 1988. Cost containment: Challenging fidelity and justice. *Hastings Center Report* 18(6):20–25.

———. 1989(a). Conflicts of interest: Profits and problems in physician referrals. *Journal of the American Medical Association* 262:390–94.

———. 1989(b). Fiscal scarcity and the inevitability of bedside budget balancing. *Archives of Internal Medicine* 149:1012–15.

———. 1989(c). Stratified scarcity: Redefining the standard of care. *Law, Medicine and Health Care* 17:356–67.

———. 1990(a). The new economics of medicine: Special challenges for psychiatry. *The Journal of Medicine and Philosophy* 15:97–119.

———. 1990(b). The law of nature and the law of the land: Of horses, zebras, and unicorns. *The Pharos* 53(2):2–6.

———. 1990(c). Physician investment and self-referral: Philosophical analysis of a contentious debate. *The Journal of Medicine and Philosophy* 15:425–48.

———. 1991. Economic disclosure and economic advocacy: New duties in the medical standard of care. *Journal of Legal Medicine* 12:275–329.

Moskowitz, A. J., B.J. Kuipers, and J. P. Kassirer. 1988. Dealing with uncertainty, risks, and tradeoffs in clinical decisions. *Annals of Internal Medicine* 108:435–49.

Moss A., and M. Siegler. 1991. Should alcoholics compete equally for liver transplantation? *Journal of the American Medical Association* 265:1295–98.

Mueller, N. 1986. The epidemiology of the human immunodeficiency virus infection. *Law, Medicine and Health Care* 14:250–58.

Mullan, F., and I. Jacoby. 1985. The town meeting for technology. *Journal of the American Medical Association* 254:1068–72.

Murray C. 1984, *Losing Ground*. New York: Basic Books.

Newhouse, J. P., W. G. Manning, C. N. Morris et al. 1981. Some interim results from a controlled trial of cost sharing in health insurance. *The New England Journal of Medicine* 305:1501–07.

Novack, D. H., B. J. Detering, R. Arnold et al. 1989. Physicians' attitudes toward using deception to resolve difficult ethical problems. *Journal of the American Medical Association* 261:2980–85.

Nutter, D. O. 1984. Access to care and the evolution of corporate, for-profit medicine. *The New England Journal of Medicine* 311:917–19.

———. 1987. Medical indigency and the public health care crisis. *The New England Journal of Medicine* 316:1156–58.

Office of Technology Assessment. 1986. *Payment for physician services: Strategies for medicare*. Washington: U.S. Government Printing Office.

Omenn, G. S., and D. A. Conrad. 1984. Implications of DRGs for clinicians. *The New England Journal of Medicine* 311:1314–17.

Page, L. 1987(a). ER physicians must provide care, but patient's plan may not pay. *American Medical News*, September 25, pp. 11, 13, 15.

———. 1987(b). Hammering out provisions both sides can live with. *American Medical News*, October 16, pp. 13,17.

Paris, J. J., R. K. Crone, and F. Reardon. 1990. Physicians' refusal of requested treatment. *The New England Journal of Medicine* 322:1012–15.

Patricelli, R. E. 1987. Employers as managers of risk, cost, and quality. *Health Affairs* 6(3):75–81.

Pellegrino, E. 1986. Rationing health care: The ethics of medical gatekeeping. *Journal of Contemporary Health Law and Policy* 2:23–45.

———. 1987. Altruism, self-interest, and medical ethics. *Journal of the American Medical Association* 258:1939–40.

Pellegrino, E., and D. Thomasma. 1981, *A philosophical basis of medical practice*. New York: Oxford University Press.

———. 1988, *For the patient's good*. New York: Oxford University Press.

Perrone, J. 1989. MD survey: Rx substitution may be harmful. *American Medical News*, May 12, p. 11.

Perry, S. 1987. The NIH consensus development program. *The New England Journal of Medicine* 317:485–88.

Pinkney, D. S. 1989. Hospital MDs facing tough times. *American Medical News* December 15, pp. 6, 7.

Platt, F. W. 1989. What do internists think? *Archives of Internal Medicine* 149:1723–24.

Platt, R. 1983. Cost containment—Another view. *The New England Journal of Medicine* 309:726–30.

Povar G., and J. Moreno. 1988. Hippocrates and the health maintenance organization: A discussion of ethical issues. *Annals of Internal Medicine* 109:419–24.

President's Commission for the Study of Ethical Problems in Medicine and Biomedical and Behavioral Research, eds. 1982 *Making Health Care Decisions*, Vol. 1. Washington: U.S. Government Printing Office.

Rainbolt, G. W. 1987. Competition and the patient-centered ethic. *The Journal of Medicine and Philosophy* 12:85–99.

Ratzan, R. M., and H. Schneiderman. 1988. AIDS, autopsies, and abandonment. *Journal of the American Medical Association* 260:3466–69.

Rawls, J. 1971(a). *A theory of justice.* Cambridge: Belknap Press of Harvard University Press.

———. 1971(b). Justice as fairness. In *Justice and Equality,* ed. J. A. Bedau, pp. 76–102, Englewood Cliffs.

Reinhardt, U.E. 1985. Future trends in the economics of medical practice and care. *The American Journal of Cardiology* 56:50C–59C.

———. 1986. Battle over medical costs isn't over. *Wall Street Journal,* October 22, p. 28.

———. 1987(a). Health insurance for the nation's poor. *Health Affairs* 6(1):101–12.

———. 1987(b). Resource allocation in health care: The allocation of lifestyles to providers. *The Milbank Quarterly* 65:153–76.

———. 1989. Health care spending and American competitiveness. *Health Affairs* 8(4):5–21.

Relman, A. S. 1983. The future of medical practice. *Health Affairs* 2(2):5–19.

———. 1985. Dealing with conflicts of interest. *The New England Journal of Medicine* 313:749–51.

———. 1986. Texas eliminates dumping. *The New England Journal of Medicine* 314:578–79.

———. 1987. Practicing medicine in the new business climate. *The New England Journal of Medicine* 316:1150–51.

———. 1988. Assessment and accountability. *The New England Journal of Medicine* 319:1220–22.

———. 1989(a). Universal health insurance: Its time has come. *The New England Journal of Medicine* 320:117–18.

———. 1989(b). American medicine at the crossroads: Signs from Canada. *The New England Journal of Medicine* 320:590–91.

———. 1990. Reforming the health care system. *The New England Journal of Medicine* 323:991–92.

Relman, A. S., and U. Reinhardt. 1986. An exchange on for-profit health care. In *For-profit enterprise in health care,* ed. B. H. Gray, pp. 209–23, Washington: National Academy Press.

Renlund, D. G., M. R. Bristow, M. R. Lybbert et al. 1987. Medicare-designated centers for cardiac transplantation. *The New England Journal of Medicine* 316:873–76.

Reuben, D. B. 1984. Learning diagnostic restraint. *The New England Journal of Medicine* 310:591–93.

Reynolds, R. A., J. A. Rizzo, and M. L. Gonzalez. 1987. The cost of medical professional liability. *Journal of the American Medical Association* 257:2776–81.

Rhodes, R. S., C. L. Krasniak, and P. K. Jones. 1986. Factors affecting length of hospital stay for femoropopliteal bypass. *The New England Journal of Medicine* 314:153–57.

Rie, M. A., and H. T. Engelhardt, Jr. 1989. The financial enforcement of living wills: Putting teeth into natural death statutes. In *Advance directives in medicine*, eds. C. Hackler, R. Moseley, and D. E. Vawter, pp. 85–92, New York: Praeger.

Riesenberg, D., R. M. Glass. 1989. The medical outcomes study. *Journal of the American Medical Association* 262:943.

Ritchie, K. 1989. The little woman meets son of DSM-III. *The Journal of Medicine and Philosophy* 14:695–708.

Robinson, J. C., D. W. Garnick, and S. J. McPhee. 1987. Market and regulatory influences on the availability of coronary angioplasty and bypass surgery in U.S. hospitals. *The New England Journal of Medicine* 317:85–90.

Robinson, J. C., and H. S. Luft. 1987. Competition and the cost of hospital care, 1972 to 1982. *Journal of the American Medical Association* 257:3241–45.

Robinson, J. C., H. S. Luft, J. McPhee, and S. S. Hunt. 1988. Hospital competition and surgical length of stay. *Journal of the American Medical Association* 259:696–700.

Roble, D. T., W. A. Knowlton, and G. A. Rosenberg. 1984. Hospital-sponsored preferred provider organizations. *Law, Medicine and Health Care* 12:204–09.

Rogers, D. E. 1986. Where have we been? Where are we going? *Daedalus* 115:209–29.

Rolph, E. S., P. B. Ginsburg, and S. D. Hosek. 1987. The regulation of preferred provider arrangements. *Health Affairs* 6(3):32–45.

Roper, W. L. 1988. Perspectives on physician-payment reform: The resource-based relative-value scale in context. *The New England Journal of Medicine* 319:865–67.

Roper, W. L., W. Winkenwerder, G. M. Hackbarth, and H. Krakauer. 1988. Effectiveness in health care: An initiative to evaluate and improve medical practice. *The New England Journal of Medicine* 319:1197–1202.

Rosenberg, C. 1983. Conflict between plan advocate and patient advocate. In *Medical Ethics*, eds. N. Abrams and M. Buckner, pp. 207–09, Cambridge: MIT Press.

Rosenblatt, R. E. 1986. Medicaid primary care case management, the doctor-patient relationship, and the politics of privatization. *Case Western Reserve Law Review* 36:915–68.

Rowe, J. W., E. Grossman, E. Bond et al. 1987. Academic geriatrics for the year 2000. *The New England Journal of Medicine* 316:1425–28.

Ruffenach, G. 1989(a). Medical tests go under the microscope. *Wall Street Journal*, February 2, p. B–1.

————. 1989(b). Premium refunds are a healthy incentive. *Wall Street Journal,* August 22, B–1.

Rundle, R. L. 1986. Some firms force employees into HMOs, and so far workers don't seem to mind. *Wall Street Journal* 10/02.

————. 1989. How doctors boost bills by misrepresenting what they do. *Wall Street Journal,* December 6, pp. A–l, A–8.

Salmon, J. W. 1987. The medical profession and the corporatization of the health section. *Theoretical Medicine* 8:19–29.

Sanders, D., and J. Dukeminier. 1968. Medical advance and legal lag: Hemodialysis and kidney transplantation. *UCLA Law Review* 15:357–413.

Sapolsky, H. M. 1986. Prospective payment in perspective. *Journal of Health Politics, Policy and Law,* 11(4):633–45.

Schaber, G. D., and C. D. Rohwer. 1984. *Contracts.* St. Paul: West.

Scheff, T. J. 1963. Decision rules, types of error, and their consequences in medical diagnosis. *Behavioral Science* 8:97–107.

Scheier, R. L. l987. Ambulatory care review seen aiding prepaid plans. *American Medical News,* April 3, pp. 2, 40.

Shertzer, M. 1986, *The elements of grammar.* New York: Collier Books/Macmillan.

Schieber, G. J., and J. P. Poullier. 1987. Recent trends in international care spending. *Health Affairs* 6(3):105–12.

Schloss, E. P. 1988. Beyond GMENAC—Another physician shortage from 2010 to 2030? *The New England Journal of Medicine* 318:920–22.

Schneider, E. L. 1989. Options to control the rising health care costs of older Americans. *Journal of the American Medical Association* 261:907–08.

Schramm, C. J. 1984. Can we solve the hospital-cost problem in our democracy? *The New England Journal of Medicine* 311:729–32.

Schroeder, S. A., L. P. Myers, S. J. McPhee et al. 1984. The failure of physician education as a cost containment strategy. *Journal of the American Medical Association* 252:225–30.

Schwartz, J. S. 1984. The role of professional medical societies in reducing practice variations. *Health Affairs* 3(2):90–101.

Schwartz, W. B. 1981. The regulation strategy for controlling hospital costs. *The New England Journal of Medicine* 305:1249–55.

————. 1987. The inevitable failure of current cost-containment strategies. *Journal of the American Medical Association* 257:220–24.

Schwartz, W. B., F. A. Sloan, and D. N. Mendelson. 1988. Why there will be little or no physician surplus between now and the year 2000. *The New England Journal of Medicine* 318:892–97.

Scitovsky, A. A. 1984. The high cost of dying: What do the data show? *Milbank Memorial Fund Quarterly* 62:591–608.

————. 1988. The economic impact of AIDS in the United States. *Health Affairs* 7(4):32–45.

Scovern, H. 1988. A physician's experiences in a for-profit staff-model HMO. *The New England Journal of Medicine* 319:787–90.

Shapiro, M. F., J. E. Ware, and C. C. Sherbourne. 1986. Effects of cost sharing on seeking care for serious and minor symptoms. *Annals of Internal Medicine* 104:246–51.

Sharfstein S. S., and A. Beigel. 1988. How to survive in the private practice of psychiatry. *American Journal of Psychiatry* 145:723–27.

Shaw, B. 1911. *The doctor's dilemma*. Baltimore: Penguin Books.

Shenkin, H. A. 1986, *Clinical practice and cost containment*. Westport: Praeger.

Shepherd, J. C. 1981. *The law of fiduciaries*. Toronto: Carswell.

Sheps, S. B. 1988. Technological imperatives and paradoxes. *Journal of the American Medical Association* 259:3312.

Shortell, S. M. 1983. Physician Involvement in hospital decision making. In *The New Health Care for Profit*, ed. B. H. Gray, pp. 73–101, Washington: National Academy Press.

Showstack, J. A., M. H. Stone, and S. A. Schroeder. 1985. The role of changing clinical practices in the rising costs of hospital care. *The New England Journal of Medicine* 313:1201–07.

Simborg, D. W. 1981. DRG creep. *The New England Journal of Medicine* 304:1602–04.

Simpson, J. A., and E. S. C. Weiner, eds. 1989, *The Oxford English dictionary*, 2nd ed., Vol. I. Oxford: Clarendon Press.

Siu, A. L., F. A. Sonnenberg, W. G. Manning, et al. 1986. Inappropriate use of hospitals in a randomized trial of health insurance plans. *The New England Journal of Medicine* 315:1259–66.

Smith, D. G., and L. Newton. 1984. Physician and patient: Respect for mutuality. *Theoretical Medicine* 5:43–60.

Soumerai, S. J. B., and Avorn J. 1990. Principles of educational outreach ('academic detailing') to improve clinical decision making. *Journal of the American Medical Association* 263:549–56.

Spicker, S. F. 1988. Marketing health care: Ethical challenge to physicians. In *The Physician as Captain of the Ship: A Critical Reappraisal*, eds. N. M. P. King, L. R. Churchill and A. W. Cross, pp. 159–76, Dordrecht: Reidel.

Spitz, B. 1987. A national survey of medicaid case-management programs. *Health Affairs* 6(1):61–70.

Spitz, B., and J. Abramson. 1987. Competition, capitation, and case management: Barriers to strategic reform. *The Milbank Quarterly* 65:348–70.

Spivey, B. E. 1984. The relation between hospital management and medical staff under a prospective-payment system. *The New England Journal of Medicine* 310:984–86.

Sprung, C. L., and Winnick B. J. 1989. Informed consent theory and practice. *Critical Care Medicine* 17:1346–54.

Starr, P. 1982, *The social transformation of American medicine*. New York: Basic Books.

Starzl, T. E., T. R. Hakala, A. Tzakis et al. 1987. A multifactorial system for equitable selection of cadaver kidney recipients. *Journal of the American Medical Association* 257:3073–75.

Stern, J. B. 1983. Bad faith suits: Are They applicable to health maintenance organizations? *West Virginia Law Review* 85:911–28.

Strong, C. 1984. The neonatologist's duty to patient and parents. *The Hastings Center Report* 14(4):10–16.

Suchman A. L., and D. A. Matthews. 1988. What makes the patient–doctor relationship therapeutic? Exploring the connexional dimension of medical care. *Annals of Internal Medicine* 108:125–30.

Swiryn, S. 1986. The doctor as gatekeeper. *Archives of Internal Medicine* 146:1789.

Tannock, I. F. 1987. Treating the patient, not just the cancer. *The New England Journal of Medicine* 317:1534–35.

Tarlov, A. R., J. E. Ware, S. Greenfield et al. 1989. The medical outcomes study: An application of methods for monitoring the results of medical care. *Journal of the American Medical Association* 262:925–30.

Thurow, L. C. 1984. Learning to say "No". *The New England Journal of Medicine* 311:1569–72.

———. 1985. Medicine versus economics. *The New England Journal of Medicine* 313:611–14.

Tierney, W. M., M. E. Miller, and C. J. McDonald. 1990. The effect on test ordering of informing physicians of the charges for outpatient diagnostic tests. *The New England Journal of Medicine* 322:1499–1504.

Todd, J. S. 1989. It is time for universal access, not universal insurance. *New England Journal of Medicine* 321:46–47.

Todd, J. S., and J. K. Horan. 1989. Physician referral—the AMA view. *Journal of the American Medical Association* 262:395–96.

United States Congress. 1989. Physician payment reform. Congressional Record 135, H-9354-H-9360 (November 21).

Veatch, R. M. 1981. *A theory of medical ethics.* New York: Basic Books.

———. 1983. Ethical dilemmas of for-profit enterprise in health care. In *The new health care for profit,* ed. B. H. Gray, pp. 125–52, Washington: National Academy Press.

———. 1986. DRGs and the ethical reallocation of resources. *Hastings Center Report* 16(3):32–40.

Veatch, R. M., and M. F. Collen. 1985. The HMO physician's duty to cut costs. *Hastings Center Report* 15(4):13–14.

Vladeck, B. C. 1984. Medicare hospital payment by diagnosis-related groups. *Annals of Internal Medicine* 100:576–91.

Waldholz, M. 1984. New views about care in hospitals lead to slower rise in health costs. *Wall Street Journal,* October 8, p. 29.

Waters, W. J., and J. T. Tierney. 1984. Hard lessons learned. *The New England Journal of Medicine* 311:1251–52.

Weithorn, L. A. 1988. Mental hospitalization of troublesome youth: An analysis of skyrocketing admission rates. *Stanford Law Review* 40:773–838.

Welch, H. G. 1989. Health care tickets for the uninsured: First class, coach, or standby? *The New England Journal of Medicine* 321:1261–64.

Welch H. G., and Larson E. B. 1988. The Oregon decision to curtail funding for organ transplantation. *The New England Journal of Medicine* 319:171–73.

Wennberg, J. E. 1987. The paradox of appropriate care. *Journal of the American Medical Association* 258:2568–69.

————. 1988. Improving the medical decision-making process. *Health Affairs* 7(1):99–106.

————. 1990. Outcomes research, cost containment, and the fear of rationing. *New England Journal of Medicine* 323:1202–04.

Wennberg, J. E., K. McPherson, and P. Caper. 1984. Will payment based on diagnosis-related groups control hospital costs? *The New England Journal of Medicine* 311:295–300.

Wennberg, J. E., J. L. Freeman, and W. J. Culp. 1987. Are hospital services rationed in New Haven or over-utilized in Boston? *The Lancet* 1:1185–88.

Wilensky, G. R. 1988. Filling the gaps in health insurance: Impact on competition. *Health Affairs* 7(3):133–49.

Wing, K. R. 1986. American health policy in the 1980's. *Case Western Reserve Law Review* 36:608–85.

Winkelman, J. W., and R. B. Hill. 1984. Clinical laboratory responses to reduced funding. *Journal of the American Medical Association* 252:2435–40.

Winslow, G. 1986. Rationing and publicity. In *The Price of Health*, eds. G. Agich and C. Begley, pp. 199–215, Dordrecht: Reidel.

Winslow, R. 1989. National health plan wins unlikely backer: business. *Wall Street Journal*, April 4, p. B–1.

Wolf, S. M. 1990. "Near death"—In the moment of decision. *The New England Journal of Medicine* 322:208–10.

Woolf, S. H. 1990. Practice guidelines: A new reality in medicine. *Archives of Internal Medicine* 150:1811–18.

Woolhandler, S., D. U. Himmelstein, B. Labar, and S. Lang. 1987. Transplanted technology: Third world options and first world science. *The New England Journal of Medicine* 317:504–06.

Wong, E. T., and T. L. Lincoln. 1983. Ready! Fire! . . . Aim! *Journal of the American Medical Association* 250:2510–13.

Yarborough, M., J. A. Scott, and L. K. Dixon. 1989. The role of beneficence in clinical genetics: Non-directive counseling reconsidered. *Theoretical Medicine* 10:139–49.

Zuckerman, S., E. R. Becker, K. Adams, et al. 1984. Physician practice patterns under hospital rate-setting programs. *Journal of the American Medical Association* 252:2589–92.

Zuger, A., and S. H. Miles. 1987. Physicians, AIDS, and occupational risk. *Journal of the American Medical Association* 258:1924–28.

CASES AND STATUTES

Becker v. Janinski 15 N.Y.S. 675 (1891).

Canterbury v. Spence 464 F.2d 772 (U.S. Ct. App. D.C. Cir. 1972).

Chew v. Meyer 527 A.2d 828 (Md. App. 1987).

Clark v. United States 402 F. 2d 950 (1968).

Cobbs v. Grant 502 P.2d 1 (Cal. 1972).

Hicks v. United States 368 F.2d 626 (4th Cir. 1966).

Meinhard v. Salmon 164 N.E. 545 (N.Y. 1928).

Natanson v. Kline 350 P.2d 1093 (Kan. 1960) reaff'd 354 P.2d 670 (Kan. 1960).

Ore. Rev. Stat Ann. 414.720, 414.725, 414.735, 414.745.

Peterson v. Hunt 84 P.2d 999 (Wash. 1938).

Pike v. Honsinger 49 NE 760, NY 1898.

Salgo v. Leland Stanford Jr. University Board of Regents 317 P.2d 170 (Cal. App. 1 Dist. 1957).

Sarchett v. Blue Shield of California 729 P. 2d 267 (Cal. 1987).

Smith v. Yohe 194 A2d 167 (Pa. 1963).

Stafford v. Neurological Medicine, Inc. 811 F.2d 470 (1987).

Wickline v. State of California 228 Cal. Rptr.661 (Cal. App.2 Dist. 1986).

Wilkinson v. Vesey 295 A.2d 676 (R.I. 1972).

Index

Access 3, 10, 22, 33–34, 47, 57, 73, 77, 85, 88–89, 91, 93–95, 114–116, 141, 143

Acquired Immune Deficiency Syndrome (*see* AIDS)

Advertising 62, 111

Advocacy 2, 71, 88–91, 93, 95, 98, 103, 110, 119–120, 125–126, 145–146

Advocate 32, 45, 88, 117, 124, 143

Aging 12, 16, 113

Agreements 72, 77–79, 83, 87, 94, 105, 107

AIDS 12, 16, 124–125

Allocation 48–50, 56, 60, 80–83, 115

Altruism 45, 51, 84, 103

Ancillary 1, 16, 28, 33, 78, 108, 117

Angina 53, 62, 75

Antibiotics 4, 49, 54, 63, 73, 92, 97, 113, 147

Assurance 49, 53, 81–82

Atomism 133, 138, 148

Atypical 70, 73

Authority 3, 29, 58–62, 64, 69, 74, 80, 89, 94, 110, 139–140, 143

Autonomy (clinical) 51, 63, 77

Autonomy (patient) 22, 46, 78–79, 104, 106–107, 114, 131–142, 146, 148

Autonomy as freedom 131–134

Autonomy as responsibility 134–138

Beneficence 46, 90

Beneficial 59, 95, 112

Benefit 10–11, 26, 33, 43, 48, 54, 56, 63, 80, 82, 88, 95, 104, 124–125, 131, 134, 145

Benefits 8–11, 24, 27, 45, 48, 54–57, 59, 63, 74, 78–79, 83–84, 90, 106–107, 111, 118, 135, 145, 147

Benevolence 80, 138

Blue Cross, Blue Shield 10, 34, 35, 52

'Boutique' health care 57

'Business class' health care 57

Business 1, 8–10, 15, 17, 22, 24, 26–27, 29, 31, 34, 44–45, 48, 57–58, 61, 104, 106, 120, 145

Buyers 21–22

Capacity (health care system) 96, 98, 109

Capacity (patient) 48, 106, 131, 134, 140–141, 145

Capacity (physician) 5, 123

Capital 9, 14, 25, 47

Capitalism 21

Capitation 25, 28, 35–36, 61

Carelessness 54, 87, 104

Case management 33

Certificate of Need 14, 25

Challenge 12, 23, 54, 58, 60, 74–75, 84, 114, 119, 126, 144–145

Challenges 6, 8, 12, 17, 21–22, 47, 51, 58, 117, 125, 148

Challenging 43, 51, 75, 78–79

Charitable 76

Charity 5, 79

Cheat 98

Chew v. Meyer 90
Chronic 11, 53, 56, 96, 125, 140
Civil disobedience 84
Clinical authority 3, 29, 58, 60–62,
     64, 69, 80, 94, 110
Clinical autonomy 51, 63, 77
Clinical protocols 52, 54, 96–97
Colleagues 31, 37, 125–127, 146
Command 63, 103
Commandeer 87, 104, 85, 88, 98,
     146
Commodity scarcity 47–50, 125
Community 8, 15, 26, 46, 77, 82, 116,
     118, 138–139, 148
Commutative justice 77
Compassion 2, 104, 142
Competing claims 2–3, 6, 64
Competing health plans, providers
     25, 27, 29, 37, 143–145
Competing interests 2, 51, 56
Competing obligations 1, 126
Competing values 5–6, 23
Competition 14, 16, 17, 21, 25–26,
     37–38, 61, 118, 143
Complex 2, 5, 38, 58, 70, 103, 109,
     139, 144, 146
Complexity 3, 44, 103–104, 139, 147
Compromise 15, 43, 53–55, 59, 70,
     76, 105, 107
Computers 11, 31, 52, 55, 64, 70, 92,
     120
Computerized tomography 9, 23, 55,
     74, 92, 113
Concurrent utilization review 32
Confidence 44, 79
Confidentiality 56
Conflict (moral) 3, 6, 51, 80
Conflicts of interest 1, 51, 60–63,
     103, 105–106, 108, 110–111,
     117–119, 121–124
Conflicts of obligation 1, 49, 51
Consensus 52–53, 95
Consent 72, 77, 104, 122, 131
Constraints 12, 17, 21, 29, 33, 37, 45,
     51, 53, 74, 112–115, 119
Construction 9–10, 14, 25
Consult 89

Consultants 30, 35–36
Consultation 22, 125
Consulting 1, 62
Consumers 21, 106–108, 143, 145
Contractarianism 45–46
Contracts 2, 27–28, 45–47, 57, 72,
     77–79, 90, 105, 116, 122
Contractual 46, 72, 77–79, 90,
     105–106, 111, 116
Contractual justice 77–79
Controls 1, 8, 11, 14–17, 24, 27–30,
     33, 37, 48–51, 53, 58–61, 63,
     69–71, 73–74, 77, 80, 86–88,
     90, 94, 98, 108, 112, 115–116,
     121,139
Convenient 76, 93
Cookbook 55, 64, 70, 127
Cooperation 29, 44, 55–56, 77, 80–83,
     89, 121, 141
Corporations 22–24, 26–28, 37, 57,
     111, 139, 142, 145
Cost-consciousness 34, 43, 108
Cost constraints 12, 37
Cost containment 13–15, 17, 22, 24,
     26–29, 31, 35–37, 43, 50–52,
     55–56, 58, 74, 78, 81, 97,
     120–122, 132
Cost effectiveness 31, 104
Cost sharing 79, 132, 144
Cost-shifting 57, 63
Costs 1, 4, 6, 8–17, 22–37, 43, 45,
     48–53, 56–59, 61, 64, 73, 76, 79,
     81, 88, 91–97, 103, 105–113,
     118–119, 122–123, 126, 132,
     137–138, 141–145, 147
Court 74, 90, 106
Covenant 45, 47
Cover 10–11, 24, 26, 33, 54, 56–57,
     73, 75–78, 109, 115, 145
Coverage 2, 11, 14, 25–26, 57, 73, 78,
     87, 89, 104–106, 108, 111, 119,
     141, 144
Covered 1, 28, 32, 77, 116
Creative writing 73
Critical minimum equivalent effort
     126
CT (*see* Computerized tomography)

Death 43, 119, 124, 135, 146
Deductibles 24, 26, 78, 107
Defensive medicine 12
Deficits 17, 23, 48, 64, 114
Denial 33, 75–76, 91, 133
Devices 15, 22, 24, 29, 32–33, 51, 73, 85, 118
Diagnosis 4–5, 15, 43, 52, 70–71, 74–75, 86, 106, 135
Diagnosis Related Groups (*see* DRGs)
Diagnostic 5, 9, 15, 26, 29, 32, 36, 52, 54, 85, 87, 94, 98, 109, 118, 137
Dictate 11, 30, 49, 55, 60, 64, 70, 147
Dignity 38, 104, 134, 137
Disability 11, 25, 43, 90, 140
Discharge 15, 32, 76, 90–92, 112, 125, 145
Disclosure 2, 104–106, 109, 111–114, 117–120, 122–123, 146
Disease 4, 10–12, 25, 48, 54, 74, 97, 119, 124–125, 137, 140
Distributive justice 77, 79–83, 91
Divided standard of care 88, 93, 103, 116, 142
DRGs 15, 25, 27, 34, 70–71, 76
Drugs 12, 21, 30, 53, 64, 109, 112, 137, 145
Dumping 57, 124
Duties 2, 46, 85–86, 88–90, 103–105, 109–111, 119–120, 131, 146
Duty 33, 44–45, 64, 72–73, 85–86, 88, 90–91, 93–95, 103–104, 106, 124, 127, 132, 139
Dyadic 1–2, 6, 139, 148

Economic advocacy 2, 88–90, 93, 103, 110, 119–120, 145–146
Economic anarchy 79
Economic disclosure 2, 104–105, 109, 117, 119–120, 146
Economic entitlements 71–73, 87, 114, 117
Education 9, 16, 26, 31–32, 50, 54, 83, 93, 145
Efficiency 21–23, 25, 51, 53–56, 59, 96–97, 115, 125, 143, 145

Efficiency guidelines 51, 55–56, 59, 97
Efficiency protocols 53–55, 96
Egalitarian 13
Elderly 4, 9–10, 12, 14, 24–25, 54–55, 57, 76, 92
Eligible 14, 21, 25, 77, 115–116, 144
Emergency 4, 30, 32, 36, 60, 92, 108–109, 111–114, 124
Employees 3, 8–9, 11, 26–27, 35, 37, 57, 61, 107, 121–122, 142, 145
Employer 77, 79, 90, 117
Engineering model of ethics 3
Entitled 13, 46, 53, 58, 73, 79, 85, 87–89, 93, 98, 105–106, 112–114, 117, 131, 137, 139, 144, 146
Entitlements 9, 16–17, 58, 71–73, 77, 79, 87, 89, 114, 117
(*see also* Economic entitlement, Moral entitlement, Legal entitlement)
Entrepreneur 16, 63–64, 93, 111, 121
Equal 3, 46, 72, 80, 83, 87, 103
Equality 57–58, 115–116
Exaggeration 71, 75
Excessive 14, 32, 38, 46, 53, 61–62, 81, 103, 107, 124, 127, 137
Expenditures 1, 8–13, 15–17, 26, 48–51, 58–59, 61–62, 85, 95, 107, 115, 126
Experimental 14, 25, 77, 145
Expertise 85, 87, 103, 116
Exploitation 44–46, 61, 63, 82, 103–106, 118

Facilities 1, 5, 9, 14, 16, 21, 25–29, 34, 36–37, 47, 60–62, 76, 86, 106, 108, 111–112, 117–118, 123
Fair exchange 58, 77
Fairness 3, 44, 46, 56, 58, 61, 74, 77, 80, 82, 115–116, 123
Faith 11, 13, 47, 82, 118
Fidelity 43–47, 51, 58, 60–61, 63–64, 69, 80, 85–88, 98, 103–104, 123–124, 131, 142

Fiduciary 6, 44, 46, 51, 58, 105–106, 146

Finances 1, 3, 8, 11, 16, 21–23, 26, 49, 120, 141, 148

'First dollar' coverage 11, 26, 105

Fiscal 2, 6, 15, 24, 27, 43, 47–51, 56, 58, 60, 63, 87, 118, 124–125

Fiscal scarcity 6, 43, 47–51, 56, 58, 60, 63, 118, 125

Flexibility 55–56, 70, 82, 92, 97

Formulary 30, 91, 112

Fraud 46, 71, 77

Free market 21–22, 138

Free rider 81–82, 143

Freedom 2, 11, 13, 30, 37–38, 45–46, 60, 62, 72, 78, 81–82, 112, 116, 122, 131–139, 141–142,148

Fringe benefits 8–9, 11, 107

Fudging 71, 75, 77

Gaming the patient 74

Gaming the system 3, 70–72, 74, 85, 98

Gatekeeper 33, 35–36

Generic 30, 35, 62

Generous 45, 47, 57, 63, 89, 144

Genetic counseling 136

GMENAC 16

GNP 8, 10, 16

Government 1, 3, 9–14, 17, 21–25, 24–26, 29, 45, 47–48, 52, 57, 61, 72, 77–79, 81–82, 107, 120, 123, 133, 139, 144

Graduate Medical Education National Advisory Committee 16

Gratuitous 45, 72, 86, 90, 93, 110

Gross National Product 8

Guidelines 51–56, 59–60, 64, 95–97, 127

Health care system 3, 6, 10, 21–24, 27, 33, 38, 47, 57, 63, 74, 81, 83, 92, 98, 114, 141, 143, 145

Health maintenance organizations (*see* HMOs)

Health Systems Agencies 14, 25

Heroism 124

HIV 12

HMOs 14, 26–29, 30, 32–37, 52, 63, 72–73, 89, 91, 107, 109, 111–112, 117, 125, 132, 142, 144

Hoard 58, 98

Honesty 2, 44, 47, 75, 77

Hospitals 1, 9–10, 14–16, 21–37, 45, 49–50, 52, 54, 57, 59, 62, 64, 70–71, 73–74, 76–77, 81, 86, 89, 91–92, 94, 107, 109–113, 117, 123–127, 133, 140

Human Immunodeficiency Virus (*see also* AIDS) 12

Hume, David 80

Iatrogenesis 53–54, 61

Ignorance 46, 106, 131, 144

Impartiality 80

Inadequacy 6, 31–32, 35, 47, 53, 72–73, 81, 94, 96, 115, 127, 131, 138, 143

Incentives 1, 10, 14–15, 24–26, 28–30, 33–38, 48, 50–51, 60–63, 81, 105, 108, 110–112, 118, 120–123, 132–133, 139

Income 35–36, 61–62, 74, 107, 121, 125, 132

Inconvenience 4, 53–54, 61, 104, 107, 126

Independence 132

Independent Practice Association (IPA) 28

Independent Practice Corporation (IPC) 28

Indigence 16, 57, 72, 74, 81, 91–94, 112–113, 123–124

Individuality 56, 64, 70, 96–9

Inequality 44, 46, 106, 116

Infantile 137–138

Inflation 10, 16

Influence 30, 44, 61, 64, 69, 80,
83, 108, 110–112, 121–123,
133–134, 138
Information 5, 21, 46, 62, 86–87, 90,
104–106, 108–109, 113–114,
118, 120, 122, 133, 135, 137,
143–146
Informed 21, 26, 62, 77, 104, 117, 119,
122, 131, 144
Informed consent 21, 77, 104, 108,
119, 122, 131, 144
Injustice 80
Inpatient 10, 26–27, 33–34, 36, 55, 73,
76, 95
Institution 25, 79, 111, 121–122
Institutional 23–24, 27, 29–33, 36–37,
43, 51–52, 59–61, 64, 94–95,
105, 109–111, 119, 121–123,
125–126, 139, 144
Institutions 1–2, 93–94, 111, 121, 123,
146
Insulate 22, 106, 132, 137
Insulation 11, 26, 31, 132–133
Insurance 3, 10–14, 22, 24, 27–29,
32–35, 52, 57, 73–75, 77–78, 84,
88–91, 98, 104, 106–107, 110,
124–127, 143–145
Insurer 28, 59, 70, 72, 74, 76–77, 89,
108–110, 113, 127, 138, 144–145
Integrity 47, 58, 77, 79, 84, 118
Intensive care 4, 43, 47–48, 50, 56, 59,
64, 75, 88–89, 107, 109, 112,
132, 136
Interests 1–2, 6, 13, 17, 21, 34, 44–46,
51, 53, 57–58, 60, 62–64, 69, 78,
80, 82–84, 86, 88, 91, 98,
103–106, 108, 110–111, 115,
118–119, 121–124, 132–133,
137, 146
Interventions 9–15, 22, 25–26, 30–33,
36–38, 48, 50–54, 58–62, 64,
69–70, 77–78, 88, 93, 95, 97,
103–104, 106–110, 113, 124,
127, 132–133, 139, 142, 145–146
Intruders 2, 134, 139
Investments 9–10, 36–37, 93,
119–121, 123

Investors 35–36, 60–62, 118, 121, 123
IPA (*see* Independent Practice Associ-
ation)
IPC (*see* Independent Practice Corpo-
ration)
Isolationism 138

Joint ventures 34
Judgment 5, 37, 55, 86, 93, 127
Justice 58, 74, 77–83, 91, 139

Law 32, 47, 58, 72, 84–86, 114–117
Legal 12, 32–33, 38, 44, 59, 71–73, 77,
79, 84, 86–87, 114–115, 117,
131, 134
Legal entitlement 72, 77, 79, 114, 117
Liability 59, 70, 86, 90, 114–117
Libertarian 13
Lithotripsy 36, 57
Litigation 34, 75
Litigiousness 12
Loyalty 13, 45, 47, 59, 105, 133

Macroallocation 50, 56
Magnetic resonance imaging (MRI)
9, 24, 36, 50, 57, 96
Malpractice 12, 34, 114–115, 117, 144
Managed care 29, 33, 48
Marginal benefit (marginal value)
54–56, 93, 98, 107
Market 3, 16, 21–22, 28, 36, 38, 57
Marketing 22, 29
Markets 21–22
Medi-Cal 25
Medicaid 9, 12, 14–15, 24–25, 72, 83,
115, 117
Medical necessity 14, 25, 32, 36, 52,
59, 64, 77, 86, 89–90, 110, 116,
126–127
Medicalization 137
Medicare 9–10, 14–15, 24–25, 27, 34,
71–72, 76, 84, 120
Metaethical 3–4
Microallocation 50

Minimum 58, 72, 80, 83, 85–86, 88,
114, 122, 126, 144
Moral entitlement 71–72, 114
Moral principles 3, 72, 83
Moral problems 3, 5–6
MRI (*see* Magnetic resonance imaging)

National Institutes of Health (NIH)
9, 52
Nonmaleficence 74
Normative 3, 5, 9, 12–13

Obligations 1–2, 6, 23, 43, 45–47, 51,
58, 63, 69, 74, 79, 85, 109–112,
114, 121, 87–88, 93–95, 98,
103–106, 121–122, 124, 126,
131, 139–142, 144–145, 148
Ontological assault 43
Outpatient 10, 15–16, 26, 28, 34, 36,
55, 73, 95, 113
Owe 2, 6, 64, 69, 72–73, 78, 85–88, 94,
98–99, 107, 109, 111, 116, 139
Own 1–3, 11, 13, 15–16, 21, 23,
27–30, 32, 34, 36–38, 43–46, 49,
51–53, 55–57, 59–60, 63–64,
69–70, 74, 77–78, 80, 82, 85–88,
91, 94, 96, 103, 106, 108, 110,
112–113, 116–118, 120–123,
127, 131–143, 145–146
Owned 1, 69
Owner 23, 61, 63

Partiality 80, 141
Paternalism 45–46, 131, 141
Payers 1–2, 6, 16–17, 22–24, 29–30,
32–33, 36, 48, 51–53, 57, 59, 64,
73–74, 77–79, 81–82, 87–88,
93–94, 96, 105–107, 108–111,
116, 118–121, 123, 125, 127, 142
Peer pressure 30–32, 62
Peer Review Organizations 14, 25
Personhood 43, 46

PET (*see* Positron emission tomography)
Philanthropy 45
Philosophy 83
Physician surplus 37
Poaching 58, 98
Policy 3, 6, 25, 36, 43, 55, 59, 73, 75,
78–79, 83–85, 88, 93–95, 107,
110, 123, 143–144
Political 9, 11–13, 44, 83–84
Positron Emission Tomography 9,
16, 48, 96
PPO (*see* Preferred Provider Organizations)
Practice parameters 51, 95, 97
Preferences 21, 56, 78, 96, 132–133,
146
Preferred Provider Organizations
26–27, 29, 34, 57
Premiums 10–11, 23–24, 35, 79, 107,
143–144
Prescribe 37, 49, 59, 63, 91
Prescription 22, 59, 77, 86, 89, 112,
139
Pressing the system 91
Prices 8, 10, 13–14, 16, 21, 27, 31, 50,
56, 59, 62–63, 69, 73, 99, 105,
107–109, 111, 118–120, 124–125
Primary care 30, 33, 35, 89
Priorities 13, 23, 51, 59, 61, 63, 78, 85,
92, 95–96, 115, 133, 148
Privacy 132
Private hospital 57, 81, 112–113
Private insurance 11, 13–14, 24, 77, 82
Private investment 9, 143
Private sector 21, 25, 57, 93, 139, 144
Productivity 12, 35, 110, 122
Profession 11, 13, 31–32, 38, 51,
87–88, 93, 96, 104, 116, 120
Professional 1–2, 5, 11, 14, 22, 25, 30,
34, 37–38, 44–45, 58, 60, 62, 69,
77, 87, 103–104, 106, 116, 118,
122–125, 131
Professional Standards Review Organizations 14, 25
Profit 16, 22–24, 27, 31, 34–35, 58, 61,
64, 107

Promises 15, 46–47, 72–73, 78–79, 90, 139
Property 22, 49, 59, 64, 85, 94, 98, 105, 107
PROs 14, 25
Prospective payment 15, 26, 48
Prospective utilization review 32, 76, 110
Prospectively 15, 109
Protect 24, 46, 106–107, 111, 133, 143
Protocols 52–55, 70, 96–97, 123
PSROs (*see* Professional Standards Review Organizations)
Purchase 13, 23–24, 30, 86, 105, 108–109, 113
Purchaser 21–22

Quality of care 3, 14–15, 21, 38, 44, 53, 58, 61, 85, 111, 122–123, 141

Rationing 25, 43, 50, 56, 80, 83, 95, 142
Reimbursement 10, 15–16, 24–26, 28–29, 32–34, 36, 38, 45, 47–48, 57, 60–61, 63–64, 70–74, 78, 86, 89, 91, 106, 110, 113, 119–120, 137
Relationship 1–2, 6, 25, 38, 44–47, 54, 72, 85, 90, 96, 104–106, 111–112, 122, 131–132, 134–135, 138–139, 148
Relative value scale 25, 120
Religious 5
Research 9–10, 12, 50, 52–54, 64, 93, 95–96
Resource policies 3, 43, 59, 88, 93, 95
Resource rules 70–71, 73–76, 79, 82, 84–85, 91–92
Resources 1–3, 6, 11, 23–24, 49, 51, 55–60, 63–64, 69–70, 72–74, 77, 80–82, 85–95, 98, 110–111, 113–114, 116–119, 121, 124–126, 133, 142, 146–147
Respect 46, 77–78, 84, 104, 131–132, 134–135, 137

Responsibility 2, 26–27, 59, 77, 90, 107–108, 110, 112, 123, 127, 134–141, 143, 146, 148
Responsible 9, 70, 107, 135–138, 140, 142–143, 148
Retrospective reimbursement 10, 15, 38, 45, 48
Retrospective utilization review 26, 32
Revenues 9, 14, 27, 29, 34–35, 43, 111, 118
Revolution 17, 64, 92, 103, 131, 138, 145, 147–148
Revolutionary disobedience 84
Right 3–4, 37, 61, 72, 83, 85, 105, 107, 114, 117, 121, 135–136, 147
Rights 2, 47, 132, 138
Risk 13, 33, 35, 43–44, 58, 104, 124, 126–127, 134, 146–147
Routine 2, 25, 36, 74, 77, 82, 88, 91, 95–96, 127, 140
Routines 15, 31, 51–52, 64, 93, 95–96

Sacrifice 5, 82, 103–104, 124–125, 127, 146
Scarce 45, 50, 56, 60, 82
Scarcity 6, 43, 47–51, 55–56, 58, 60, 63–64, 73–74, 80, 114, 116, 118, 125
Service 10, 27–28, 30, 36–37, 44–45, 58, 81, 86, 106, 108–109, 115–116, 121, 141–143
Services 1, 10–11, 15–16, 21–22, 25, 27–29, 32–34, 60–61, 72, 76–78, 91, 94, 103, 105, 107–108, 115–116, 120–121, 123, 143–144
Shaw, George Bernard 44
Simplistic 3, 63, 69, 86, 88, 104, 123, 139
Skill 1, 45, 63, 85–87, 103–104, 126
Skillful 13, 44, 87
SME (*see* Standard of Medical Expertise)
Societal 38, 43, 83, 93
Society 2, 6, 12–13, 17, 45–46, 50, 52, 56–57, 59, 64, 73–74, 78, 80,

Society (*continued*) 83–85, 87–88, 93, 97, 108, 116, 121, 127, 132, 134, 138, 148
SRU (*see* Standard of Resource Use)
Stafford, Pauline 74–75
Standard of care 16, 56–57, 85–88, 93–94, 103, 113–116, 142
Standard of Medical Expertise 87, 103, 116
Standard of Resource Use 87–88, 93, 98, 103, 116–117, 142
Standardization 51, 54, 64, 92, 95–96
Sticker shock 109
Stockholders 49, 80, 107
Stratified scarcity 51, 56, 58, 64, 73–74, 114, 116
Subsidization 81

Tax Equity and Fiscal Reform Act (TEFRA) 15
Taxpayers 49, 80, 107
Technologies 1, 9, 12, 14, 23–25, 27, 29, 34, 36, 47, 49, 57, 59, 61–63, 72, 86, 95, 103–104, 116, 139
Technology 9–11, 13–14, 23–24, 50, 92, 98, 104
TEFRA (*see* Tax Equity and Fiscal Reform Act)
Tests 9–10, 14–16, 35–36, 49, 52, 54, 59, 71, 73, 75, 78, 97–98, 107–108, 115, 125–126, 132, 137, 140
Therapeutic substitution 30
Therapy 4, 29, 53–54, 59–60, 71, 109
Third parties 43, 54, 71, 134
Tiers 51, 57–58, 114

Traditional 2, 6, 15, 23, 27–30, 43–44, 47, 50–51, 58, 60–61, 64, 69, 73, 80, 85–88, 90, 98, 103–104, 123, 131, 138, 144
Transplant 13, 25, 30, 48, 50, 56
Treatment 5, 10, 26, 43–44, 54, 95, 106, 107–109, 113–115, 119–120, 123, 133–134, 144–146
Trust 13, 44, 58, 75, 85, 106, 118, 121

Unbundle 10
Uncertainty 3, 5, 13, 31, 51, 53–54, 96–98, 109, 122–123
Uncompensated care 57, 74, 81, 111
Uncompensated costs 59
Uncompensated debt 76
Uninsured 78, 114
UR (*see* Utilization review)
Utilization review 29, 32–34, 48, 52, 62, 70–71, 73, 75–76, 88, 91–92, 110–111, 122–123, 126–127

Value 5, 13, 22, 25, 27, 31–32, 51, 54–55, 93, 97–98, 107, 120, 132, 135–136, 141–142, 145, 147
Values 3–6, 12–13, 38, 46, 48, 54, 56, 60, 76, 78, 80, 83, 96–97, 104, 106, 134–136, 142, 146–148
Veracity 74, 76, 89, 104
Virtue 31, 45, 47, 104
Vulnerability 13, 43–46, 58, 63, 85, 104–106, 118, 131–132, 140, 146

Witchcraft 85